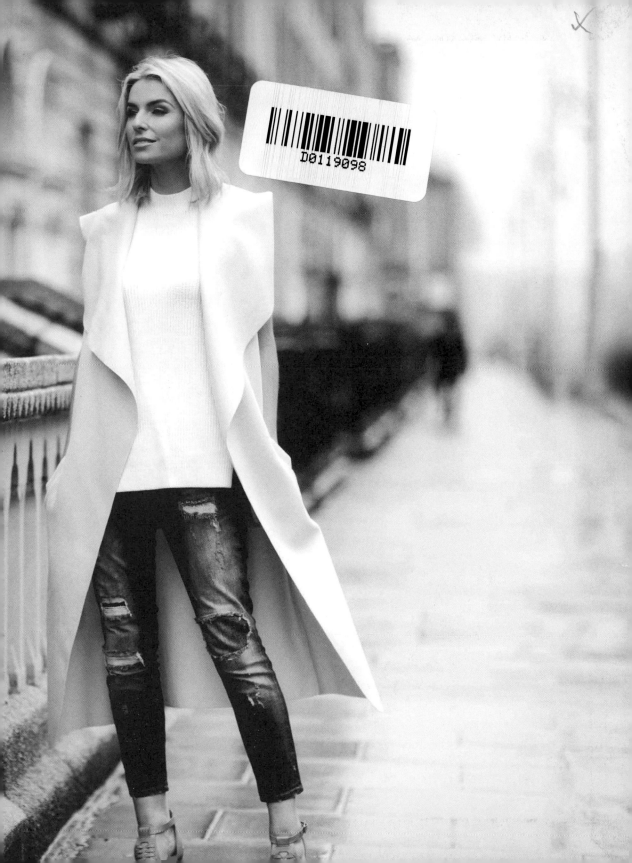

PIPPA

PIPPA

SIMPLE TIPS TO LIVE BEAUTIFULLY

PIPPA O'CONNOR

PENGUIN

IRELAND

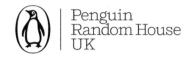

Penguin
Random House
UK

PENGUIN IRELAND

UK | USA | Canada | Ireland | Australia
India | New Zealand | South Africa

Penguin Ireland is part of the Penguin Random House group of companies
whose addresses can be found at global.penguinrandomhouse.com.

First published 2016
001

Copyright © Pippa O'Connor Ormond, 2016
The moral right of the author has been asserted

Typeset by Perfect Bound Ltd
Printed in China

A CIP catalogue record for this book is available from the British Library
ISBN: 978–1–844–88378–3

www.greenpenguin.co.uk

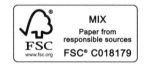

MIX
Paper from
responsible sources
FSC® C018179

Penguin Random House is committed to a
sustainable future for our business, our readers
and our planet. This book is made from Forest
Stewardship Council® certified paper.

Picture credits

All © Lili Forberg except:

pp. 5, 10, 34, 35, 46, 51 (tl, mr, bl & br), 67, 78, 79, 88, 115, 135, 137, 153 (all), 157, 162–3, 168–69, 173, 276 (tl, tr & br), 280–81, 284–5, 288 (tl, tr & br) and 302 Pippa O'Connor Ormond.

p. 7 Mark Stedman/Photocall Ireland.

p. 33 and 136 Brian McEvoy.

Shutterstock: p. 28 WorldWide; p. 55 (mr) www.BillionPhotos.com; p. 55 (tl & bl) imtmphoto; p. 105 Rido; p. 106 liewluck; p. 107 gpointstudio; p. 112 Gayvoronskaya_Yana; p. 119 Andrey_Popov; p. 120 Letterberry; p. 121 Maxsol; p. 125 vitals; p. 129 Pontus Edenberg; p. 133 (tl) Picsfive; p. 133 (tr) Nataliia K; p. 141 Julenochek; p. 142 Tania Zbrodko; p. 143 Kae Deezign; p. 149 Svetlana Lukienko; p. 151 wanpatsorn; p. 166–7 Dmitry Zimin; p. 166–7 Everything; p. 190 Lena Ivanova; p. 192 Grigor Unkovski; p. 193 MaraZe; p. 204 Andrey_Popov; p. 205 Robert Przybysz; p. 227 (tr) Alena Ozerova; p. 227 (bl) Odua Images.

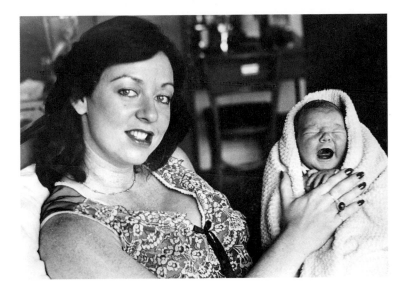

For my beautiful mum, Louise.
Our guardian angel.

CONTENTS

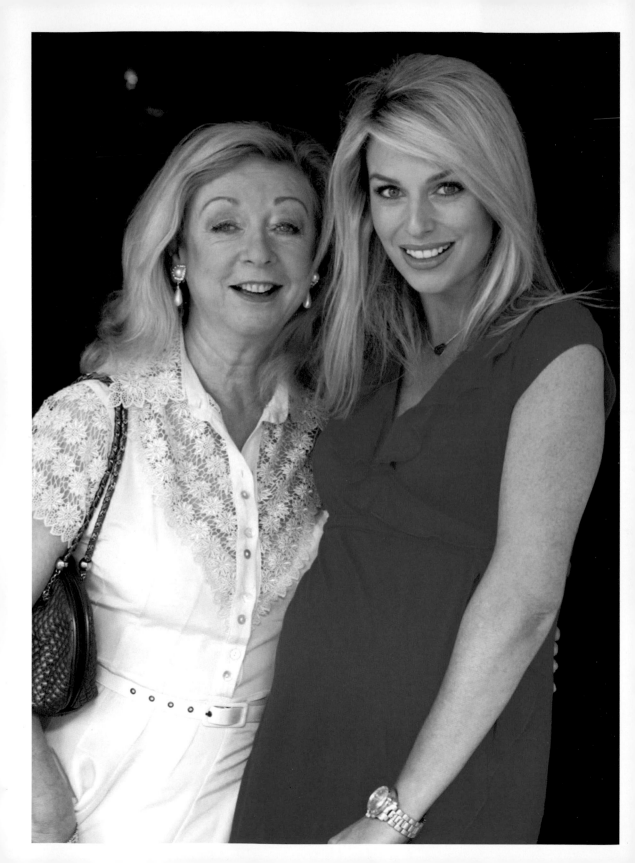

INTRODUCTION

Like most little girls I always loved to play dressing-up. I would go into my mother's room, put on her red lipstick and jewellery and picture myself as a grown-up as I posed in the mirror.

My mum, Louise, was the epitome of style and sophistication, always with her hair freshly blow-dried and nails painted red. She trained in Paris as a cordon bleu chef when she was young. She ran her own restaurant and then a catering company when I was a small baby. She worked hard back then. Working in a kitchen is far from glamorous but she would do it in pencil skirts and high heels as if that was normal. She used to tell me stories how she'd often have to bring me to the kitchen in my Moses basket as she worked.

When it came to fashion, she had an old fashioned way of thinking. She believed in dressing appropriately for the occasion. You would never see her going into town shopping in her trainers. ('Trainers are for the gym, are they not?') She could never understand why I wore trainers and ripped jeans. That was just her!

My mum taught me so much about fashion, style and interiors. She was a massive influence, without me even realizing it at the time. She had a great eye for everything from decorating to flower arranging. You know when someone just has the touch and makes everything look effortless? Well, that was her.

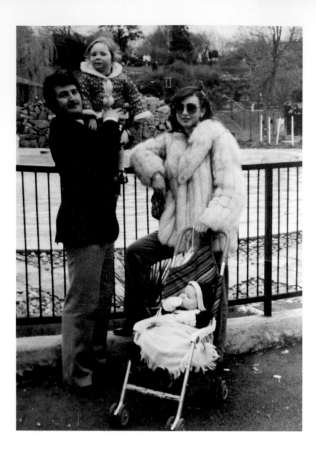

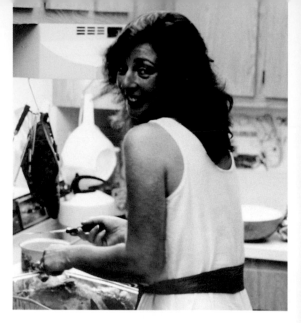

LEFT *My glam mum at Dublin Zoo with my brother Cian in the buggy and Dad holding my sister Susanna.*
ABOVE *Mum in the kitchen.*
RIGHT *With my husband Brian and our son Ollie.*
FAR RIGHT *Me in the kitchen.*

She would host dinner parties on a regular basis when we were children. For most people, the thought of cooking a three-course meal, arranging the house to look like something out of a Laura Ashley book and entertaining your guests would leave you in a cold sweat. But to her it came naturally, and that's what she loved.

Tragically, my beautiful mum passed away very suddenly on 11 October 2014, aged only sixty-one. I miss her dreadfully, especially now as I write this book. She would have adored this and got such a kick out of it.

I'm the youngest of three. I have a sister, Susanna, and brother, Cian. Susanna is six years older than me, so when we were young that felt like a huge gap. I envied her clothes and all of her nice accessories. I would take her things without asking, which of course resulted in

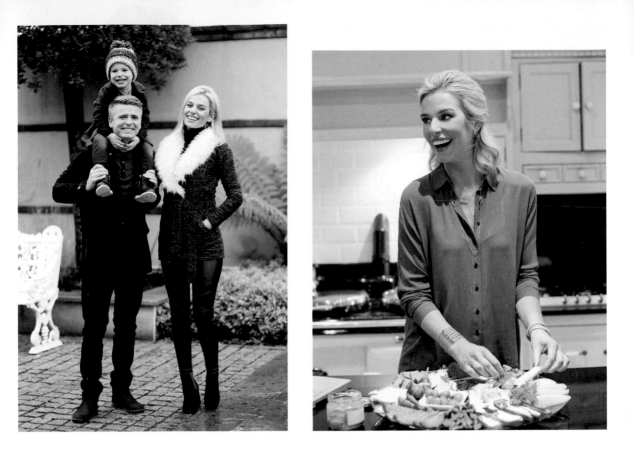

massive arguments. She even resorted to putting a lock on her wardrobe when she went travelling, which I managed to open! Now we are both in our thirties, we're the best of friends. The tables have turned since our childhood and she's the one taking my things these days.

To me, anybody can be stylish, regardless of money, age or body shape. I don't believe you need to spend a fortune to look and feel fabulous, far from it. Style is about using your imagination and feeling confident in your skin. If you don't feel good on the inside, it'll show on the outside.

I haven't always felt so confident when it comes to fashion. I've been through lots of years of dodgy hair, over-plucked eyebrows, bad clothes and too much fake tan!

However, the older I've become, the more confident I am in my own skin. I think it's since I became a mother, too. I'm way more relaxed and sure of who I am. I don't follow trends that I know won't suit me and I've learned to make the best of what I have.

During my ten years of modelling, I also picked up some amazing tips and tricks. It wasn't all glamorous though – far from it! I had years of driving up and down the country in my Fiat Punto at all hours of the day and night going from job to job. For some early morning TV slots I'd literally have five or ten minutes to get ready – and I'll tell you how to do that in the book, don't worry!

I loved my modelling years and it certainly paved the way for where I am today but I was never really fulfilled. It was only after having my son, Ollie, in 2013 that I knew I wanted to share my passions, which were fashion, beauty and interiors. So I set about creating pippa.ie, a website where I give daily updates on my outfits, fashion loves and finds, as well as my beauty secrets. Within a year, pippa.ie blew up and it's now one of the most popular website destinations in Ireland for women to get their daily updates.

In 2014, my next project was born when I created a face and eyeshadow palette with the help of fellow businesswoman and friend Una Tynan, founder of Blank Canvas Cosmetics. The Pippa Palette – consisting of six warm to medium matte eyeshadows, a highlighter, a blusher and a bronzer – was released in the summer of 2015. Originally planned as a limited edition, the Pippa Palette became such a success that we've continued to keep it rolling. To this day, it blows my mind seeing so many women using and enjoying a product that I created.

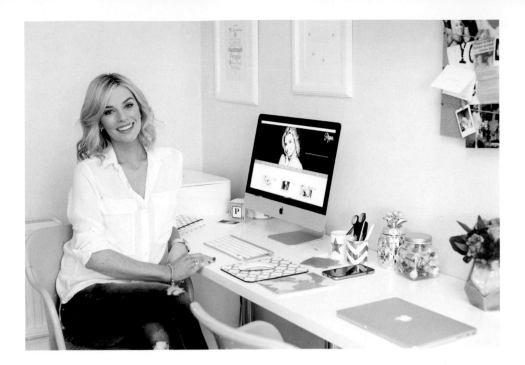

So, now that I run a business as well as being a busy mum, I thought I'd share the tips and techniques I've learned along the way. My aim was to write a book full of useful and simple information, such as how to get ready in ten minutes, the essential items every woman needs in her wardrobe, what to wear to a wedding, how to travel in style (and with kids!), easy ways to create a beautiful home, and how to be the perfect hostess!

This book really is for everyone – as anyone can be stylish! – so I really hope you'll enjoy my Simple Tips to Live Beautifully.

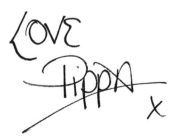

PART ONE: FASHION

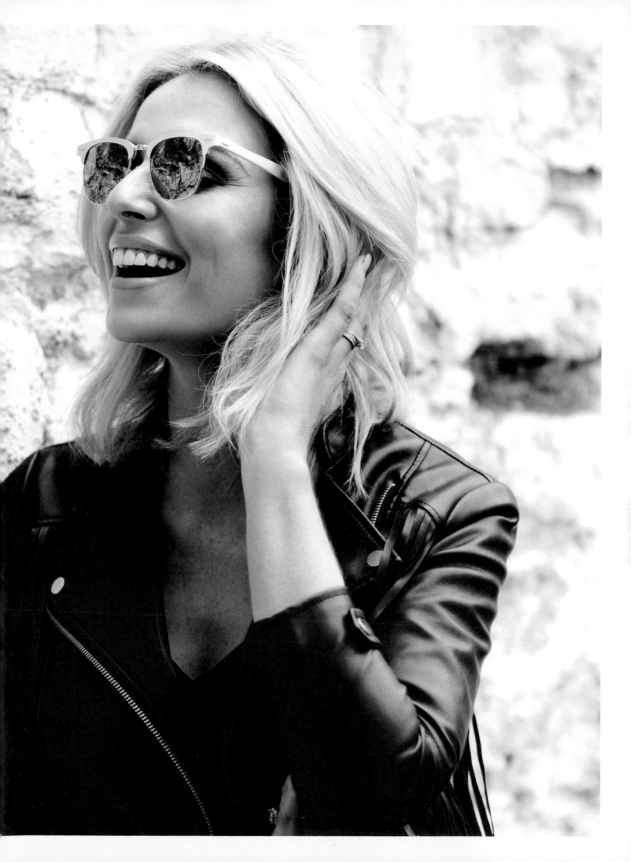

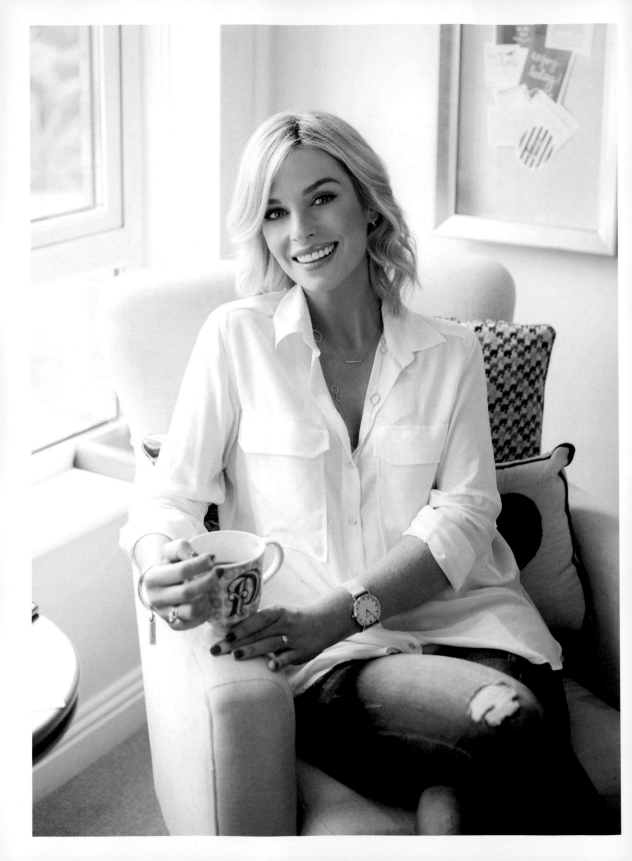

CHAPTER ONE

YOUR STYLE: THE BASICS

Everyone has their own style and taste – whether you realize it or not, people are always attracted to similar things. To me, being stylish is mainly about confidence. It's about wearing what you love and not buying something just because it's in fashion or it looks good on someone else. Sure, it's great to keep up with the trends and know what's popular, but that doesn't mean you must follow suit. I love keeping up-to-date with catwalk trends but I don't necessarily go out and buy similar versions. I take elements of things I'm inspired by to help me create my own style.

It's taken me a long time to find my own style. I never had the confidence before now to wear what I love. It's easy to buy what the magazines are showing us or to copy our friends. So, how do you get the confidence, you might be thinking?

Well, firstly you need to accept who you are. Accept your height, shape and boob size, and have a good look at your body to determine your shape first of all. If you know your body-type, you're halfway there to feeling and looking fabulous.

It's all about proportion and helping your proportions look their very best. Always focus on shape and silhouette instead of height and weight. Each of us is unique and our bodies are too. Love what your mother gave you, and dress for what you are now, and not what you wish you were. Nevertheless, our body shapes are generally narrowed down to four categories. You may find that you fall into two categories, in which case you can take elements from each to work for you.

APPLE

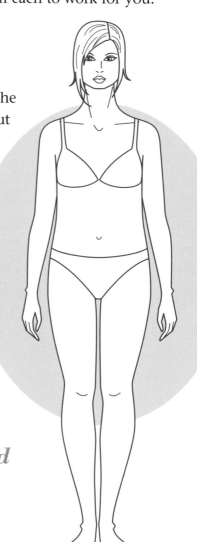

Most of your weight accumulates above the hips, which are narrow, so you tend to put weight on your belly.

- Draw attention to those legs as they are your best asset.

- Go for shorter skirts with tops that are slightly fitted, but wear soft and lightweight fabrics.

- Wear loose fitted shirts with sleeves rolled up, teamed with skinny jeans and killer heels.

You're in good company with Drew Barrymore and Reese Witherspoon.

HOURGLASS

If you have the Marilyn Monroe-esque figure, count yourself lucky. Having an hourglass figure means you're well proportioned on top and bottom and have a defined waist.

- Accentuate your curves by showing off your waist.

- Choose clothes that follow the natural curves of your shape, instead of hiding it.

- Go for low to medium neck lines that accentuate the bust and balance out the hips.

- V-necks and scoop necks are great too.

- A-line and pencil skirts hug your curves in all the right places and look fab with a fitted top.

- Avoid boxy jackets or shift dresses.

You're in good company with Marilyn Monroe, Kelly Brook and Kim Kardashian.

RECTANGLE

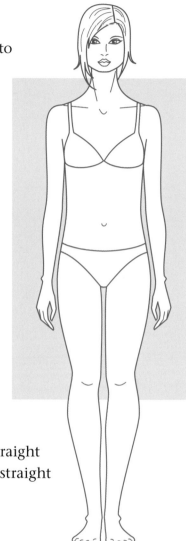

Probably the easiest shape when it comes to finding clothes, as your bust and hips are more or less the same width and you generally have lean legs and a slim straight frame.

- You can really wear what you like… oversized tees, jumpers, floaty dresses.

- You can opt to create the illusion of curves by sporting pieces with certain details like a chunky belt around the waist.

- Boyfriend jeans, cropped or tailored trousers will look great with flats.

- Asymetric dresses will accentuate the curves on your body.

- Avoid wearing pieces that all have straight lines from head to toe, for example, straight blazer, straight jeans, straight tee.

You're in good company with Cameron Diaz and Nicole Kidman.

PEAR

Your lower body is broader than your upper body.

- Layering on your top half creates visual interest and draws the eye upwards.

- Your jackets and tops should finish either above or below the widest part of your hips and bottom.

- Mid-rise jeans are most flattering.

- Have fun with colour and striking necklines.

- Kimono and bell sleeve tops will really flatter.

- Best to avoid details, patterns or pockets on your thigh and hip area.

You're in good company with J-Lo, Beyonce and Shakira.

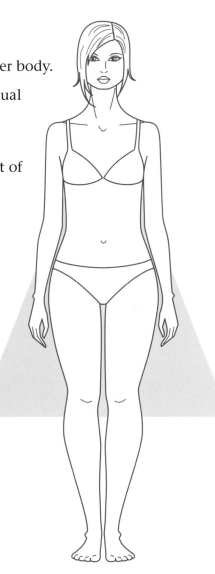

GET INSPIRED

Once you've got the basics sorted and understand which kind of clothes and shapes suit you, start thinking about the styles you love. Get creative and really think about what inspires you and the kind of look you're after.

I get my inspiration from everyday women walking down the street. I love to people watch. My favourite thing to do is to sit outside a cafe – in the summer months especially – and watch the world go by! I love looking at what women are wearing.

Social media is another huge source of inspiration. I adore Instagram and enjoy following fashion bloggers from all over the world. I love seeing bloggers' street style too. Pinterest is also a great source for ideas and inspiration – I strongly advise you get the app!

Magazines also give me good ideas. Even if the price tag is too high, I'll take bits and pieces of an outfit that catches my eye and adapt it to my style – and budget! I admire lots of celebrities' style too, like Olivia Palermo and Blake Lively – they're two of my favourites. Both are very polished but constantly take fashion risks, which I love!

Your personality should shine through with your clothes and choices. So, when it comes to creating your own style, try to be open-minded and never be afraid!

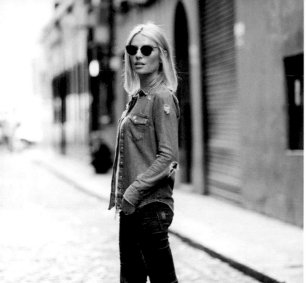
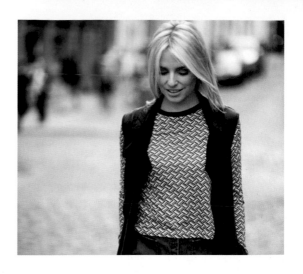
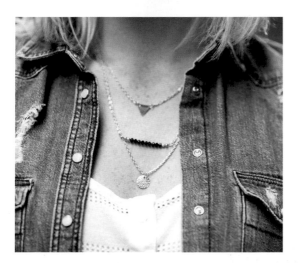
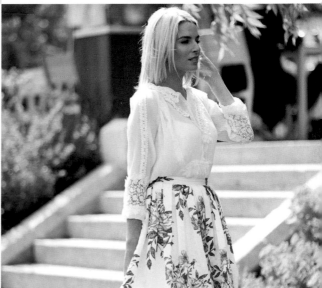
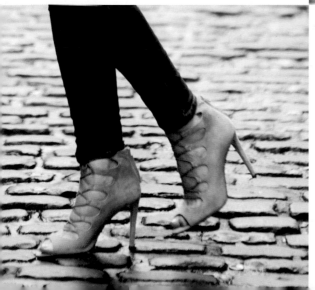
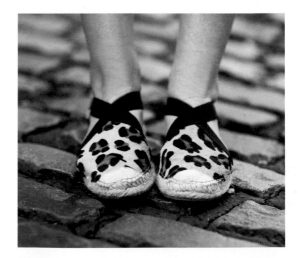

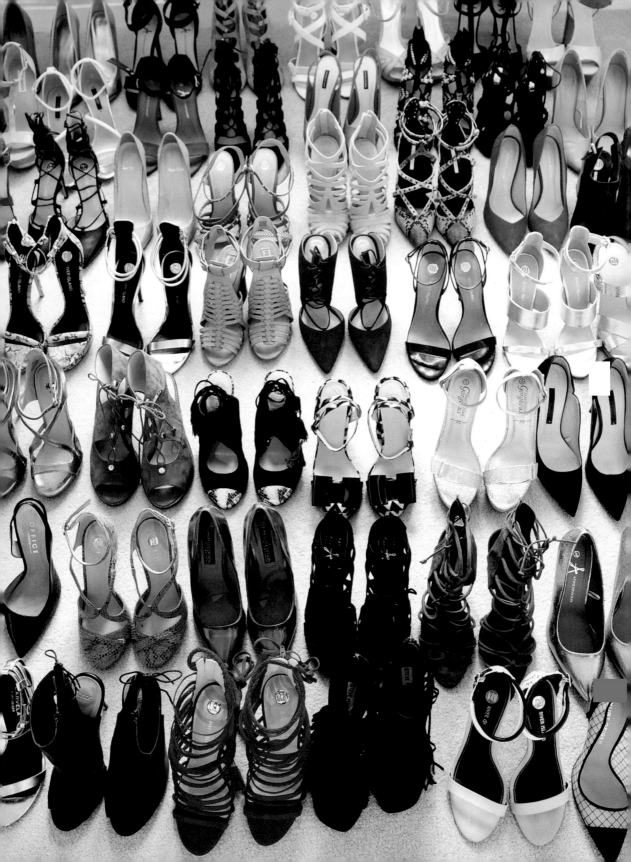

DETOX YOUR WARDROBE

Before we talk fashion, I recommend a detox. When I say detox, I don't mean on yourself, I mean on your wardrobe! I'll admit I'm not the most naturally organized person in the world when it comes to my clothes – but I have taught myself to be. This is essential for lots of reasons. First, I find it stressful going to bed with a mountain of clothes on the chair and the wardrobe bulging with items I don't even wear. Second, I end up buying clothes I already have, or had forgotten about, just because I couldn't see them clearly. Now, I detox at least twice a year – and this means going through every drawer and item in the wardrobe. So, ship your kids off, or just take a full day to yourself, put on your favourite music and pull everything out.

BE RUTHLESS . . .

These are the seven deadly sins, all lurking deep at the back of our wardrobes. For wardrobe nirvana, this is a good place to start.

- If you haven't worn something in 8–12 months, get rid of it. You aren't suddenly going to wear it again. The exception to the rule is if you're pregnant and you're not going to be back in your regular clothes for at least a year.

- If it's too small, don't keep it. Don't torture yourself by thinking I'll fit into that some day.

- The same goes for shoes, if they're too big or too small, or they've really just had their day, or you're like a newborn giraffe walking in them – they need to go too!

- If anything is damaged or beyond repair get rid of it also.

- White tops and shirts that have gone off colour or have tan marks need to go.

- The same applies to white underwear that is discoloured – you'll never feel amazing in them if they've gone grey.

- Handbags and accessories – obviously hang on to good pieces as you'll have them forever and they usually wear well, but say goodbye to anything cheap and cheerful that is tarnished or tatty looking. Wearing a ring that makes your finger go black isn't going to get you any style points!

. . . BUT DON'T BE TOO RUTHLESS!

Obviously, rash decisions can lead to regrets later on, so remember these points before you get too carried away.

- Hold on to classic items, like a good plain black dress, a tailored coat, a black blazer – these don't go out of fashion.

- Be creative. A blazer, for instance, might feel a little boring or dated but if you changed or added amazing gold buttons think about how it would look then.

- Do you have an old bridesmaid's dress or wedding guest outfit that could be revamped or cut? Look at everything very carefully before making decisions.

DIVIDE ITEMS INTO DIFFERENT PILES

Pile one: bin
For anything that's broken or unwearable.

Pile two: charity
Clean and wearable, but not right for you anymore.

Pile three: sell
I've tried Depop before and found it great.

Pile four: friends
Invite friends over and show them your unwanted items before you give any away.

SPACE

How much space do you have in your house? Do you have lots of it or do you need to think about storing winter clothes over the summer and vice versa?

No matter whether you store your clothes under your bed, in a spare room or in your attic, make sure you do this in a neat and organized way. Put your items into a sealed see-through plastic box (Ikea have these). Clearly label what they are, for instance maternity clothes, winter knits or summer beach wear.

Once you know what space you're working with, it's time to put everything back neatly and in order. Before you do that it's a good idea to give your wardrobe and drawers a good clean and a dust down. Now is also a good time to line your underwear and sock drawers with some scented drawer liners.

HOW I ORGANIZE MY CLOTHES

- I keep my going-out, more glam clothes, like tops, dresses, leather trousers, etc, in my hanging space. I try not to layer clothes on hangers as it's easy to forget what's underneath.

- Hang your everyday clothes, like casual tops, shirts, cardigans, skirts, trousers or work clothes, where they're most visible and you can easily get to them as you'll probably be reaching for these most often.

- On my shelves, I keep my jeans and heavier knitwear.

- In my chest of drawers, starting from the bottom up, I keep pyjamas, then tanning clothes, followed by lounge/fitness wear followed by t-shirts/cami tops. In the top drawers, I keep underwear, socks and tights.

- Occasion-wear, such as dresses for a wedding, I keep in a wardrobe in the spare room. Some of these I keep in a garment/dry-cleaning bag so that they're protected from dust.

- And for my shoes, I have an amazing shoe wall, built by my very own husband, which you can see on page 257. You can also use shoe racks or even plastic or canvas shoe pockets which you can hang in or on the side of your wardrobe or on the back of a door. For long boots, insert a shoe tree as this will help to keep their shape and keep them looking good for longer.

WHAT'S MISSING?

Now that you're organized and can see what you have, it's good to make a list of what you're missing. Your list should consist of timeless key items that won't go out of fashion, then you can add to your wardrobe with trend-led items like a printed blazer or a fringed skirt.

HOW TO LOOK SLIMMER

No matter what your shape, it's important to look streamlined. Here are some invaluable tips to help you look slimmer:

Shapewear

Shapewear is so, so important. Even if you're slim, it's good to have a smooth silhouette. Spanx and other stretchy devices have been around for years now – made even more popular by British stars Trinny and Susannah. They work extremely well to smooth you out and hold you in in all the right places. I think Marks and Spencer has an excellent selection of shapewear.

The right bra

Having the correct bra is just as important. It's so crazy the number of us women not wearing the correct bra size! I myself have gone for bra fittings in the past only to be told I'm a completely different size to what I thought. So, take yourself to a good department store that offers a free bra-fitting service. You'll be amazed how much better your clothes will look and fit once you're in the correct size. Not to mention appearing slimmer. And if you've had children or are pregnant, remember your size is going to yo-yo.

Stand tall

When you slump, you literally lose inches in your height. When your body is in alignment, your head is sitting squarely on your shoulders and your shoulders are pulled back with your core muscles pulled in, you increase your height and stretch out your body mass. Not only does this make you look thinner, but you're also projecting an image of confidence.

Show some skin

Expose a bit of skin with a V-neckline. The open, upside-down triangle creates a high focal point up and away from your midsection and gives the illusion of a longer, slimmer upper body. The more skin displayed between chin and chest (within reason!), the more elegant your proportions will seem overall. Wider V-necklines also visually balance broad hips and thighs.

Slimming shoes

Choosing shoes that have a low-cut vamp will instantly elongate and slenderize your leg. A vamp is the portion of a shoe that cuts across your foot at the front. So, a low vamp cuts across the base of the toes, while a high vamp would come up the foot or possibly to the ankle. A nude shade of shoes will elongate your legs even further.

HOW TO LOOK GREAT
IN A PHOTOGRAPH

This is something we all want to perfect and that doesn't just apply to models. Social media is taking (or has taken!) over the world and everyone loves sharing beautiful pictures of themselves – and why not, I say! I have a few simple tips that will help you get the very best picture of yourself. Here's what I do:

- If you're posing with a group of three or more people, try standing on the outside. I'll let you in on my vain secret, I always stand to the left of the other person. I just feel the left hand side is my better side! I sound crazy now, don't I? Or do you all have 'a side'? My poor husband just knows the drill now and knows what side he should be on to suit me!

- Always stand slightly at an angle, never front on, as it's just not as flattering.

- Stand tall, with your shoulders back.

- Slightly point out your leg, so for me it would be my left leg if I'm standing on the left-hand side.

- Keep your face slightly tilted at an angle, and ever so slightly stretch so you elongate your neck. You won't look like an ostrich, I promise!

- Keep your tongue at the roof of your mouth; this will help disguise any double chin.

- Keep your eyes wide open, without looking like a rabbit in the headlights. As Tyra Banks would say, 'smize' (smile with your eyes).

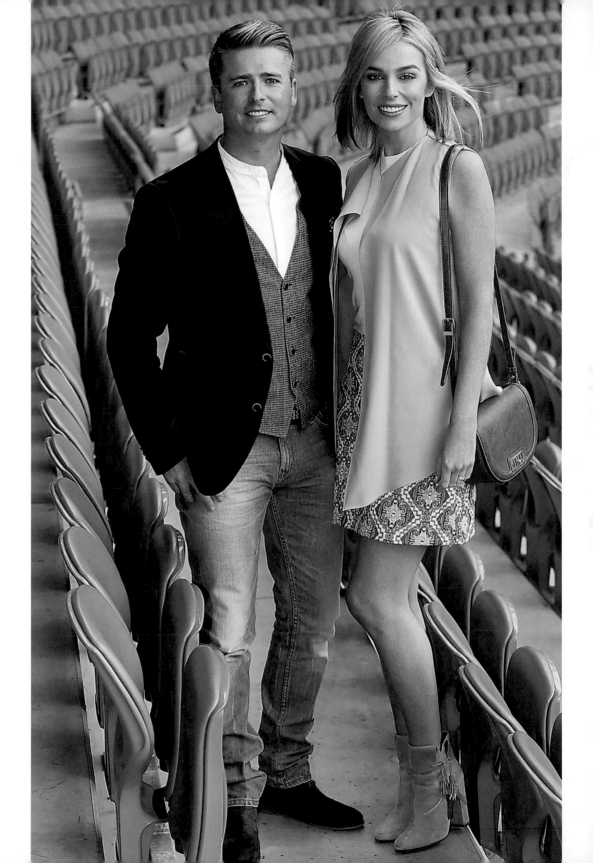

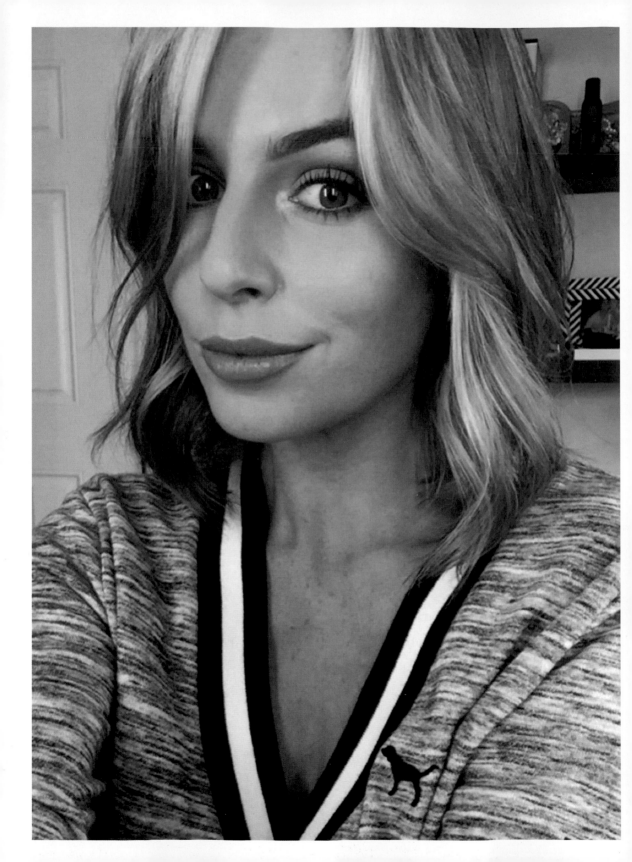

HOW TO TAKE A SELFIE

It's a question I get asked a lot: 'How do you take a decent selfie?' I've taken a fair few in my time, so I think I've perfected how to look my best at this stage.

- When it comes to selfies, light is key! Go to a window. A frosted window in a bathroom works really well. You want the light to hit you from the front, not from behind.

- Hold your arm higher than your face, it's more flattering from a height.

- Again tilt your head to the side, chin slightly angled down.

- Tongue to the roof of your mouth or mouth open if you want to show off your teeth.

- Eyes wide open but don't overly lift your eyebrows or you'll just look shocked.

- Proceed to take a hundred selfies until you're happy!!

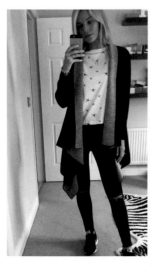
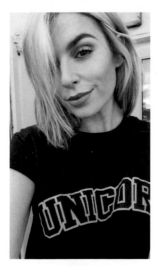
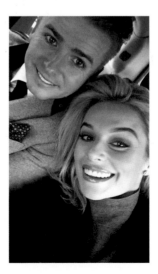

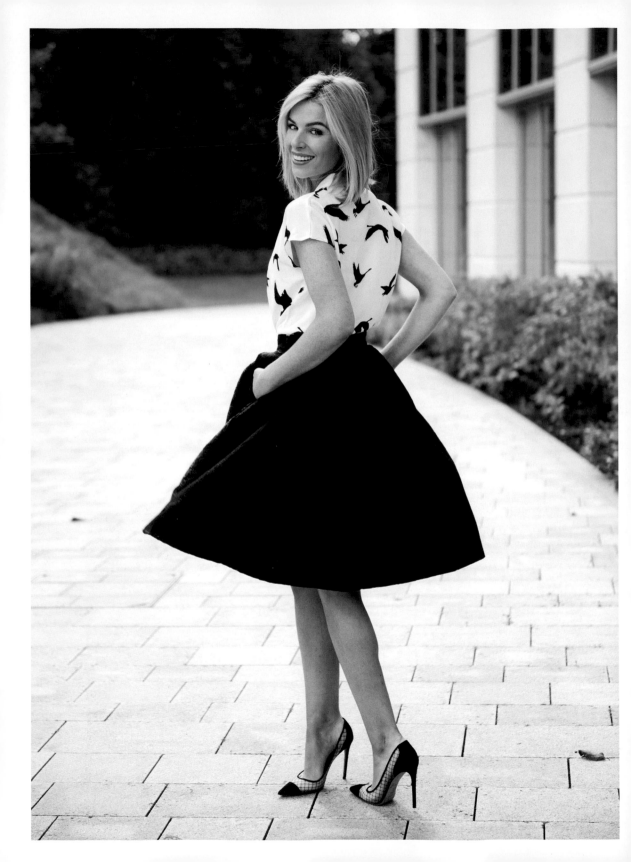

CHAPTER TWO

WHAT TO WEAR

I don't think there should be any 'rules' when it comes to fashion. I truly believe that if you love something, you should wear it! It's that simple. If you love something – and it suits you and your shape, and you feel good in it – wear it!

A lot of women email me every day asking for advice on what they should wear to certain occasions, beauty product recommendations and lifestyle advice. A wide range of age groups follow me, anything from teens to sixties. One thing I've been asked time and time again is, 'Am I too old to wear that?' Very recently, a woman in her mid-forties emailed me to say how much she loves fashion and takes lots of inspiration from things I post on pippa.ie (brilliant, I'm thinking!). However, she said most of her friends and colleagues dress a lot older than her, even though they're a similar age, and should she being doing the same? What's appropriate and what's not? She wanted to know my opinion.

I replied, reminding her of a few well-known and stylish ladies who are near the same age but breaking all the rules. Heidi Klum, forty-two, and J. Lo, forty-six, to name but two. I told her that if she loved something, wear it. Who says you can't wear leather trousers when you're sixty? Hello, Christie Brinkley! Most thirty-year-olds would be envious of her style.

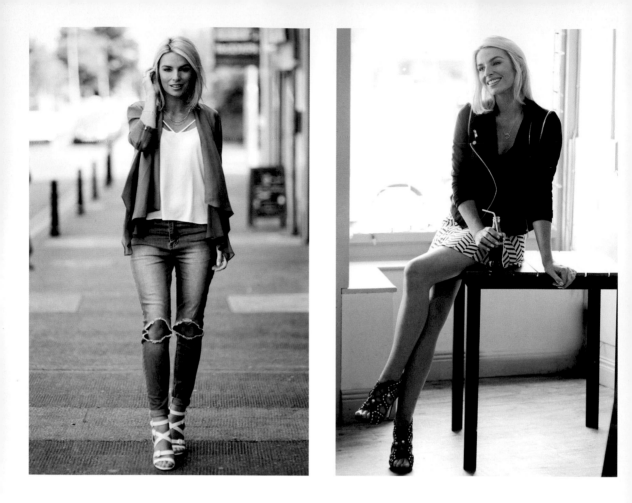

It's not about age, it's about dressing appropriately and knowing your shape. Personally, I don't like showing off legs and cleavage at once, but that goes for a sixty-year-old as much as it does for a twenty-year-old. I love getting my pins out because I'm confident in short hem lines, but if I'm doing that I'll go demure on top with a high neck and long sleeves. It's good to leave some things to the imagination.

So, I don't believe in following rules as such. Just be sure that what you're wearing fits and flatters you and, most importantly, walk with confidence. By following that one rule, you'll be able to rock anything – no matter what age you are!

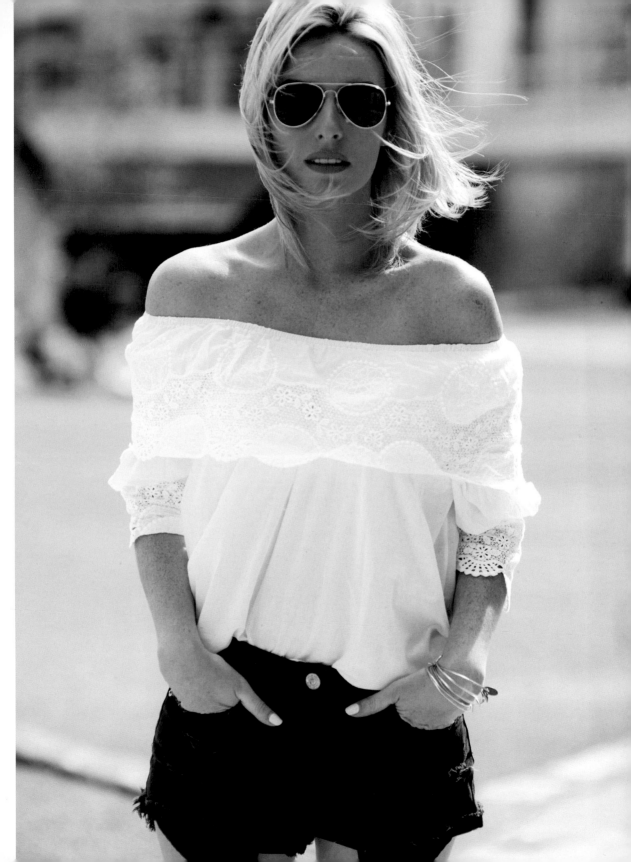

THE ESSENTIALS

So, what are the essential items that make up an ideal wardrobe? For me, it's the following:

Black leather jacket

When spending money on a good leather jacket, my advice would be to go for a classic style rather than one particularly on-trend with either fringing, studding or a cropped style. A classic jacket will see through each season and you can always buy faux leather if you want to follow a certain trend.

LBD

Never underestimate the little black dress, it can literally take you to any occasion. When investing in this, I would go for something classic, well fitted and plain. This means you can then accessorize it to suit any occasion.

Jeans

I know it can be really hard to find your perfect pair (I'll tell you how to do that in a minute!) but once you do, these will remain a staple in your wardrobe for many years to come.

Basic t-shirts

You should have some really good quality t-shirts in black, grey and white. I have wasted money before buying cheap ones, which really don't hold their shape or wash well. I believe when you buy cheap, you buy twice. You will wear them on their own in summer, layered under knits, blazers or denim shirts. As well as wearing casually, you can also wear your t-shirt with tailored trousers and a statement necklace for a cool, edgier look.

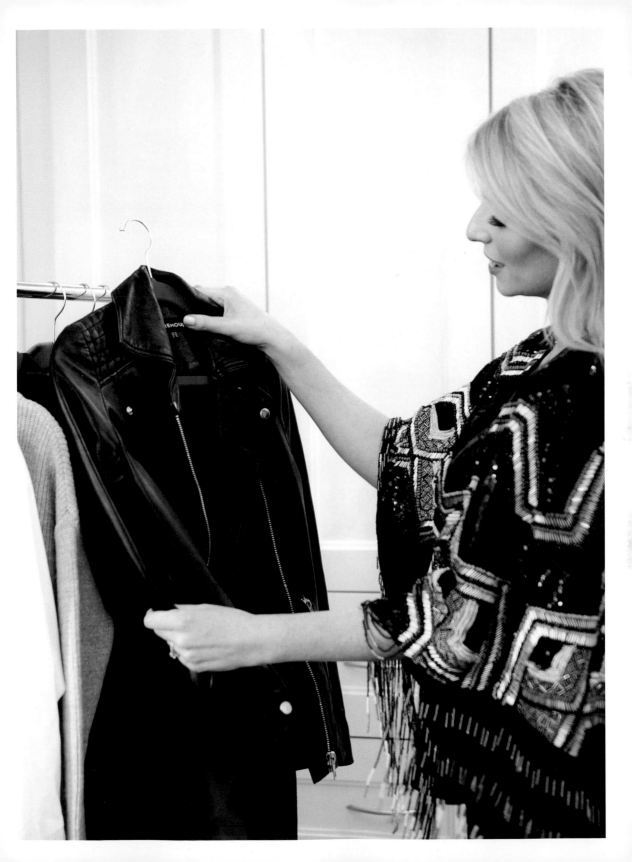

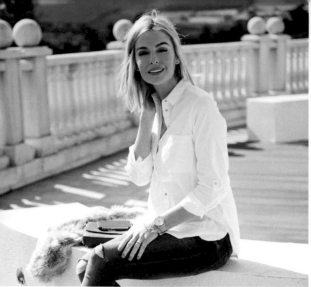
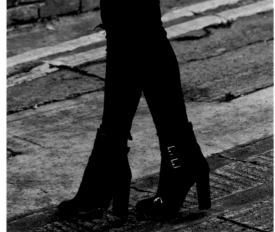
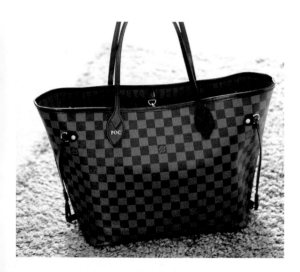
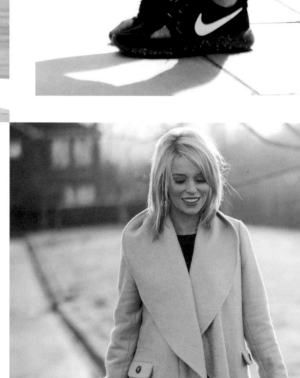
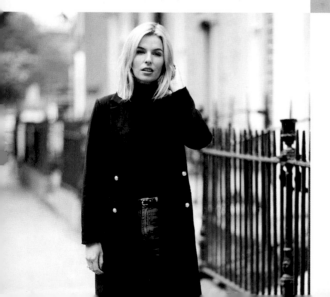

White shirt

This should be a casual loose fit. I think white shirts look great with sleeves rolled up and the top buttons undone, teamed with any pair of trousers or jeans – it's a really great look.

Tote bag in black or tan

A good tote bag will see you through everything from work to weekend wear.

Boots

I probably get most wear out of my black ankle boots. As a busy mum, I want to be comfortable but look stylish, and I can be both in flat ankle boots or a block-heeled boot.

Trainers and slip-ons

A must for everyday wear and for easy comfort when travelling.

Black coat

It's an obvious one but so essential. So much so, that I probably own ten 'essential' black coats in a variety of styles. A black coat will take you absolutely anywhere. It's smart, even with boyfriend jeans and trainers. Or, over any dress, a black coat just pulls your outfit together instantly.

Camel coat

A woollen camel coat reminds me of my mum or granny. It's such a classic. The camel coat has become so popular again. It's never really gone out of fashion but you see them all over the high street right now. Camel looks amazing over a cream turtle neck. That's one of my favourite colour combos. I have a great sleeveless camel coat too, and I love layering underneath it. I'll wear a plain tee and open denim shirt under it.

HOW TO SHOP FOR JEANS

Let's be honest, most women probably dread shopping for jeans. There are so many brands and styles to choose from, and even when you know your right size it's difficult to know if a pair will suit you.

The only way around this is to try them on in the store. You need to go jeans shopping with that sole purpose in mind. It's important to have a few good pairs that fit you well. A pair of perfect, figure-hugging jeans are a staple item and can form part of any outfit from casual to dressy.

THE FIT

When trying on your jeans they should feel tight, unless you're going for a relaxed boyfriend fit. I don't mean uncomfortably so, but you should have to bend your knees and jump up again to get into them. If they go on too easily and you can fit your whole hand down the back of them, then they're too big.

Jeans will loosen, and look and feel better the more you wear them.

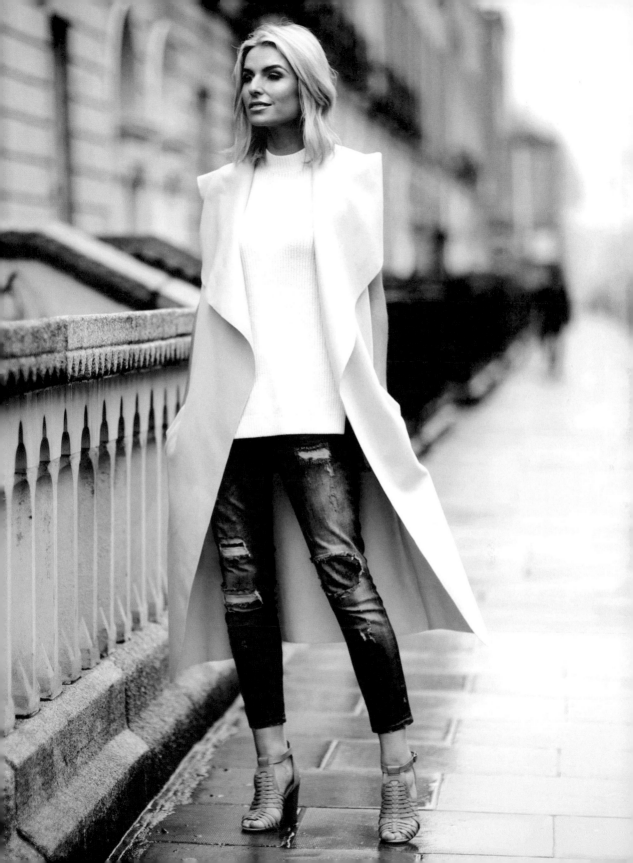

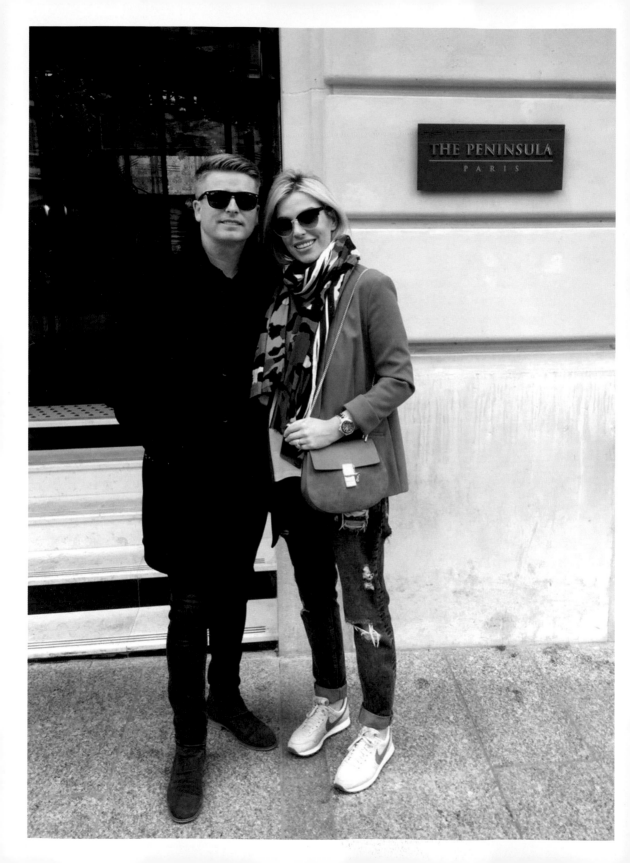

Skinny jeans

One of my favourite styles. They look super day or night with flats or heels. High-wasted skinny jeans are great if you want to show off your curves. I go for a really soft denim when buying skinny jeans.

Flared jeans

Go for a seventies vibe in flared jeans. They've become so popular again. I think they look amazing. The bell-bottom shape makes you look taller and can make your thighs and waist appear smaller.

Boyfriend jeans

These roomier, loose-fitting jeans look great on lots of body types. They look effortless and cool on slim women but equally they look super on curvier hourglass figures. I love wearing mine with my Nikes and I usually turn them up slightly – teamed with a tight fitting top and loose blazer. It's a look I love!

Low rise

Probably best on women with a flat stomach as they sit quite low under your belly button.

Mid rise

These will look great on everyone, really, as they sit just perfectly at your belly button.

High rise

I have a friend who's the perfect pear shape and high rise look incredible on her. She has curves in all the right places with a small waist and they just look so sexy and slimming.

TOP TIPS FOR JEANS

- If buying white or cream jeans, do not go for ones that are a struggle to get into. For example, I'm usually a size 8 in jeans but when I buy cream (personally, I prefer cream rather than white), I buy a size 10. They look awful if they're too tight or see-through. Make sure they aren't see-through!!

If you're self-conscious in jeans always opt for a darker denim as they are slimming and will make you feel more confident.

- When jeans shopping, take a pair of heels with you. If you are buying a boot-cut or flare take the highest heel you have, so you can judge if the length will then work with a slightly lower heel.

- Ask a sales assistant – many of them can offer good advice and know their stuff when it comes to denims.

- It's best to wash your jeans as little as possible. When you do, make sure they're inside out and in a cool wash. Air dry them.

- Small pockets make your bum look bigger. Big pockets make your bum look smaller.

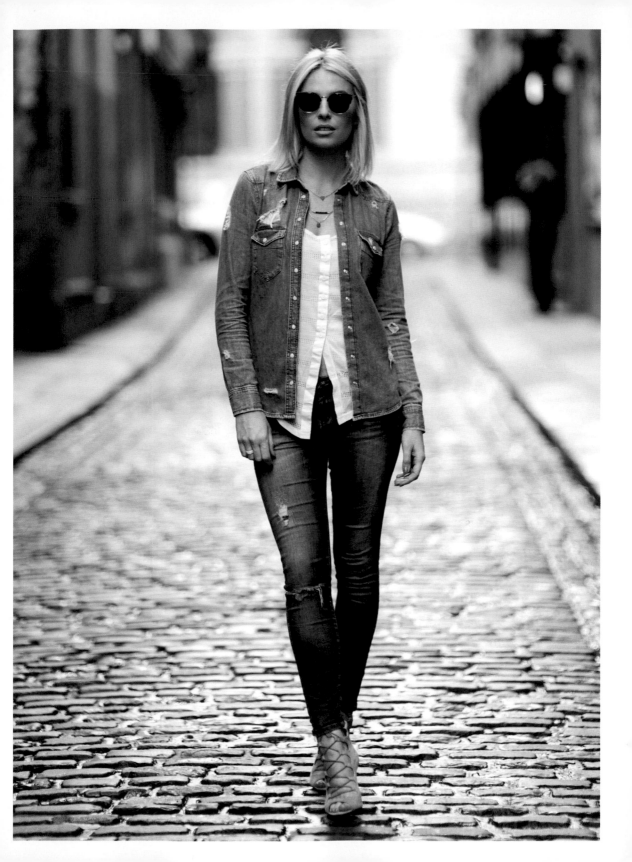

HOW TO UP-STYLE AN OUTFIT

So you're a little bored of your existing outfits and hear yourself saying 'I've nothing to wear' – you know, the usual! You could always adapt and accessorize some basic items in your wardrobe and – ta da! – you have a new outfit!

- Take your favourite pair of jeans (you could even rip these slightly at the knees, if you're into that) and an old oversized knit. Feels a little dull?

- Okay, so now roll up the sleeves and tuck one side of your knit into your jeans.

- Gather up some gold bangles. If you have none, go to Penneys/ Primark or H&M, they have brill jewellery to jazz up any outfit. Stack them high on one of your wrists, add a delicate gold chain.

- Tie your hair in a high ponytail. Choose some bold killer heels.

- Pop on some bright lippy and instantly you'll feel fabulous in your old outfit.

When it comes to updating an old black dress or a plain black top and shorts, you simply need two or three items to reinvent the outfit. A belt for the dress, maybe an obi belt that will cinch you in at the waist, or a satin belt encrusted with beading would look fab. For the top, just add a statement necklace, then pick a cool pair of heels, clash with a leopard-print clutch, and you have a chic nighttime look.

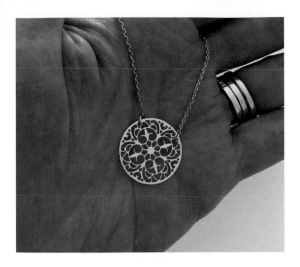
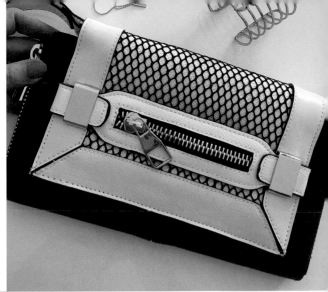
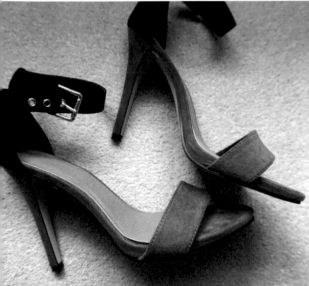
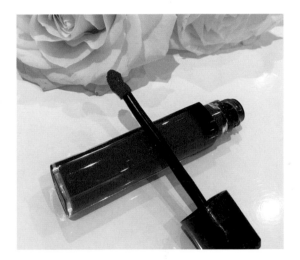
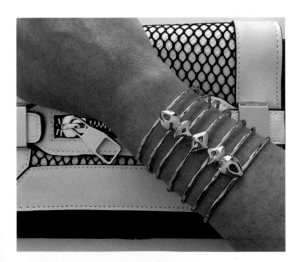
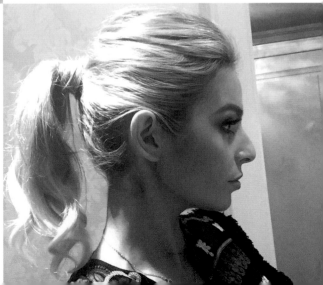

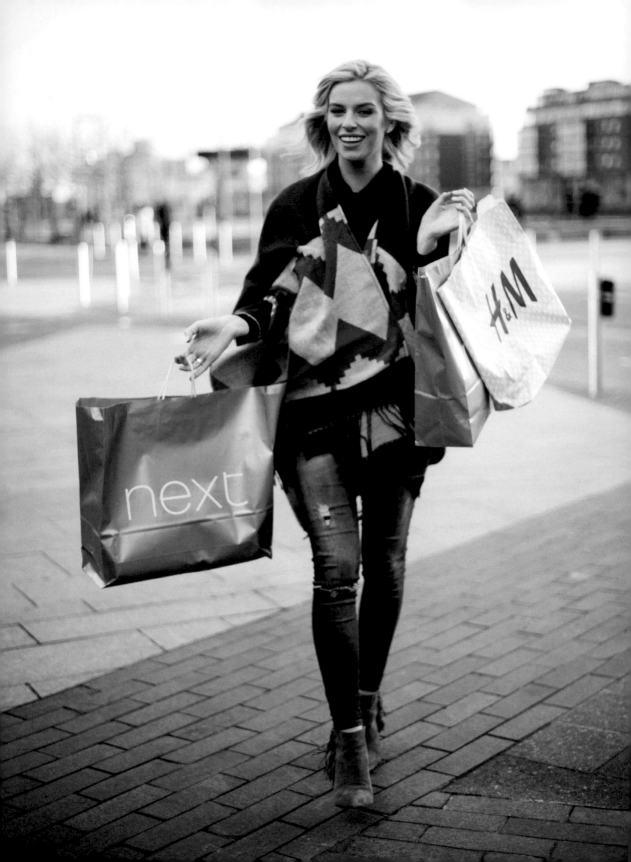

HOW TO SHOP THE SALES

I love a good sale. There's nothing more thrilling than getting something really fabulous at a bargain price. What I don't like about sales are the queues, the mess and the crowds. Sales such as Black Friday or the January sales can also make us lose the plot a bit and we end up buying something just because it's at an unbelievable price. But don't panic, here are are my top tips on how to beat the sales *and* get what you want without all that fuss.

- Look at what you have in your wardrobe and write out a list of things you're missing. Preferably staples, like a designer bag or black jacket.

- Do some research before you hit the shops. Go and look in your favourite places. Sales assistants will often tell you the exact day the sale is starting, or it'll be advertised. Try on things now, know your size and earmark them for later.

- Don't buy rubbish. Don't waste your money on something you'd never love enough to pay full price for just because it's on sale.

- Don't go for slogan tees or sequinned tops. These aren't 'good buys' as they often go out of date quickly.

- Set yourself a budget and don't go over it. I've been there, it's too easy to get over excited, especially when you see 70% off!!

- Try things on if you're not sure – don't make a guess – and wear flattering underwear that'll suit most things you try. Wear comfortable loose clothing and flat shoes that are easy to slip on and off. Bring a small-sized crossover handbag so that your arms are free.

Leave your other half and kids at home! This is an important one.

When you're on a mission like sale shopping, it's best to go alone.

- Perhaps buy one really good piece instead of five more jumpers and two more tops!

  Recently this is what I did around Black Friday. I really wanted a pair of over-the-knee black suede Stuart Weitzman boots so I held off until the sales hit, put my blinkers on and headed straight to the shoe department knowing what I was looking for. I got €200 off! Fabulous! They were still expensive but that's all I bought and they're something I absolutely love.

- Sales are a great time to buy designer bags or shoes. If you've always dreamt of a Mulberry bag, now's the time to get it. It's easier shopping for shoes and bags in the sales too.

- Look online. Often sales start earlier online, so keep a close eye on them. They can sometimes offer a bigger discount too.

- Don't be fooled by very old stock. I've worked in retail, back in the day when I was in my late teens, and I didn't know what I wanted to do with my life! I loved meeting people and this really taught me how much I loved fashion and helping people choose outfits.

  Back to my point though! Often shops will drag really old stock out to get rid of it. So you could be tricked into buying something that's years old just because they want to clear their stock rooms.

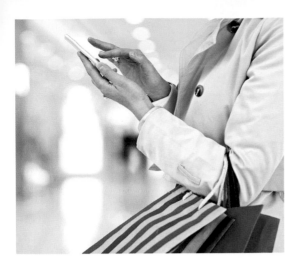
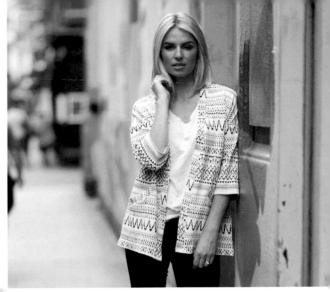
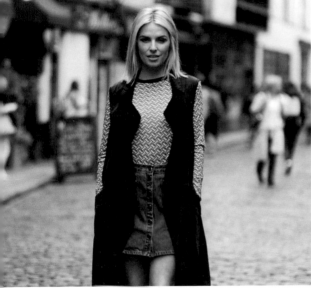
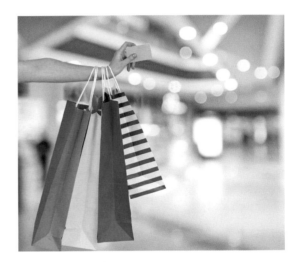
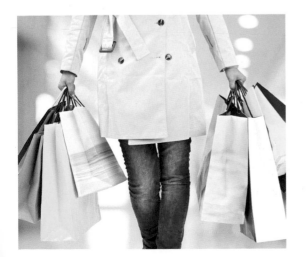
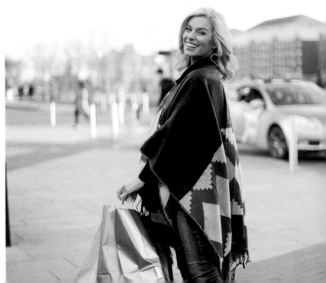

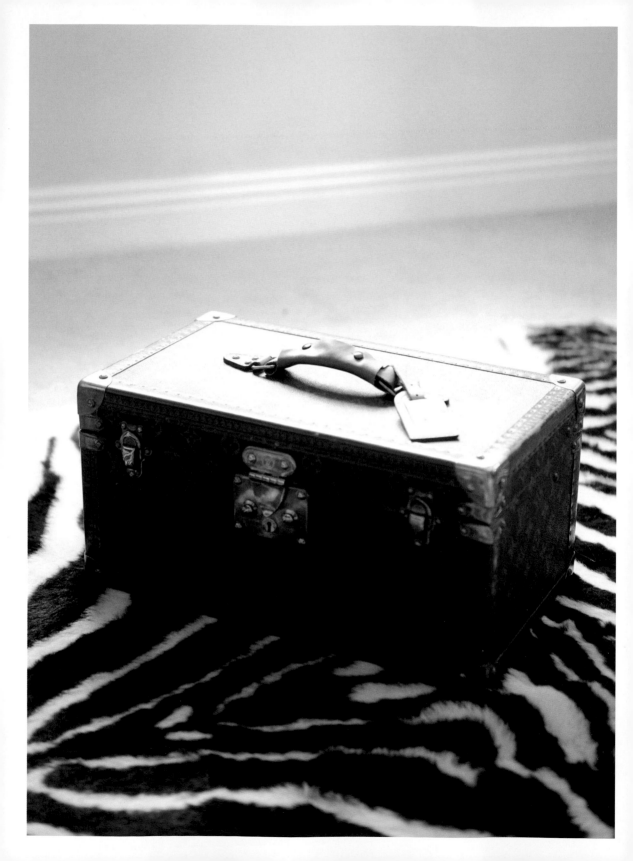

BUYING INVESTMENT PIECES

I love the way we call them 'investment' pieces like we're going to get some return on them. We're not. Unless you sell them at a profit, which is unlikely. But it sounds better and makes you feel better about spending above normal budget on some items. Saying that, if you are going to wear something again and again, you could argue it's well worth paying that bit more.

So when spending a month's rent on an 'investment' piece, it's important to make sure you're purchasing wisely.

Investment pieces shouldn't be too trendy. They should consist of some classics like a cashmere sweater or scarf. A good pair of sunglasses, a suede or leather jacket. Classic boots, like my Stuart Weitzmans. Or a good coat.

When I was about nine years old my mum brought me to London for the first time. Just the two of us. She had just turned forty and was obviously treating herself, and me, to a shopping spree. I was blown away by London and especially by Harrods – the children's toy department was like something I'd only ever seen in the movies. To this day, I love going in there and thinking about that first time. It's still just as magical.

On our last day, and after being treated to some toys in Harrods, we were making our way back to the airport in a black cab. My mum told the driver to pull up and let us out. We were at Louis Vuitton. She told me that she had had her heart set on something for a long, long time, and today was the day she was going to treat herself.

As soon as we entered the shop she knew what she was looking for. It was the large hardsided vanity case. She bought it without hesitation. Not that she could afford it, but still, she clearly wanted it so got it anyway. It weighs a ton and is totally impractical for travelling but, oh my God, is it beautiful to look at!

Every holiday or night away she insisted on bringing her pride and joy. She'd laugh and say it was her favourite thing so she would use it. I loved it and once told her I wanted one when I was grown up. She'd often joke and say, 'Philippa, that's yours when I'm gone.' (She was the only person ever to call me by my full name. Never once did she call me Pippa.)

So, obviously, I now have her beloved Louis V case. It still looks perfect and smells like new. To me, that's an investment! To have something like that that you can pass down is special and something to be treasured.

When you're going to make a big purchase, do it wholeheartedly. You could make some memories and, without sounding morbid, leave something beautiful behind.

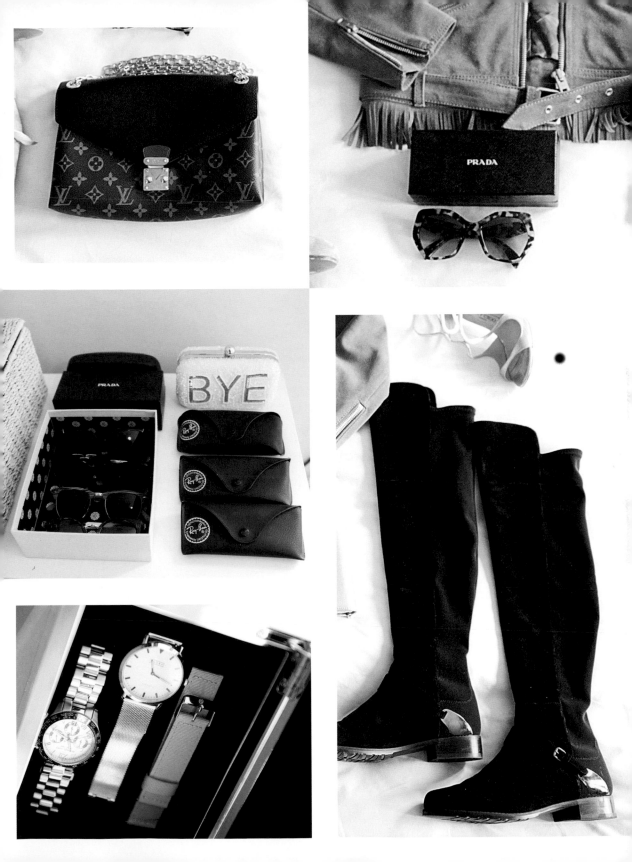

HANDBAGS

I think my love of handbags started as a little girl. I was obsessed with looking at my mum's collection and rooting through the contents. A handbag just made me feel like a grown-up. I also loved the look of handbags stored together neatly on a shelf. All so different, in all sorts of colours, shapes and sizes.

A handbag is something that you can always use. Even when I'm sporting baby bumps my trusty handbags are still my friends! They can pick up the plainest of outfits, change a whole look and generally just take your outfit to another level.

I actually don't spend much money on expensive clothes. Yes, I've treated myself to some special designer pieces over the years but, in general, I'm a high street girl. Handbags, though, are probably the one thing I'm most likely to spend money on. So, if you're going to splash out, save up or ask Santa nicely, here are a few things to consider:

- Is this bag practical? Think about what you're going to use it for. If it's a clutch bag for evening wear, make sure you test it out. Does it fit your phone, lipstick and other small essentials? If the answer is no, it's probably not worth spending that much money on. Sorry!

- Will the bag wear well? It's good to consider whether the material in your bag is going to scratch or stain easily.

- Is it comfortable? I love chain bags, but some are killers on your shoulders and just aren't comfy. If the bag is really big, will it be too heavy to carry around all day? Think about your posture and back!

- Textured leather will wear better and is easier to care for than satin or suede.

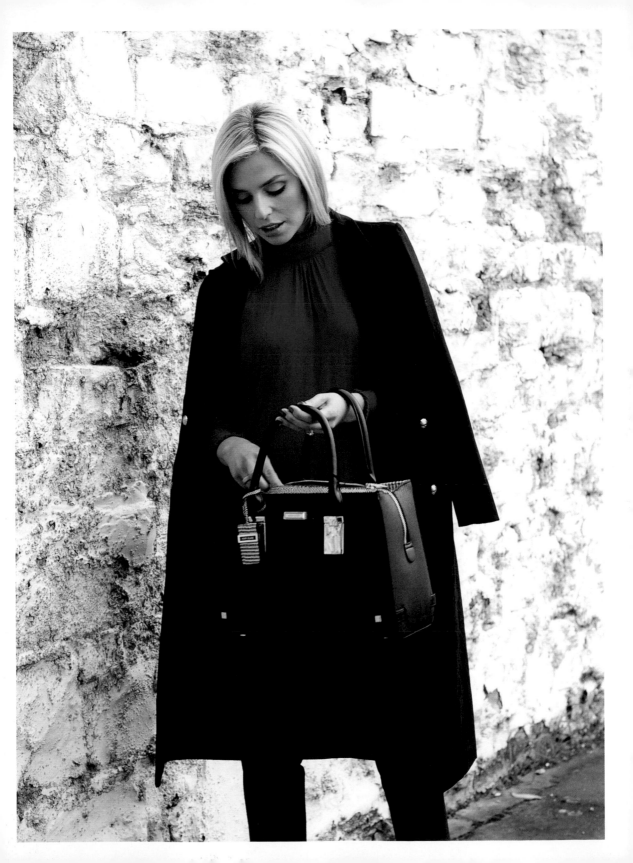

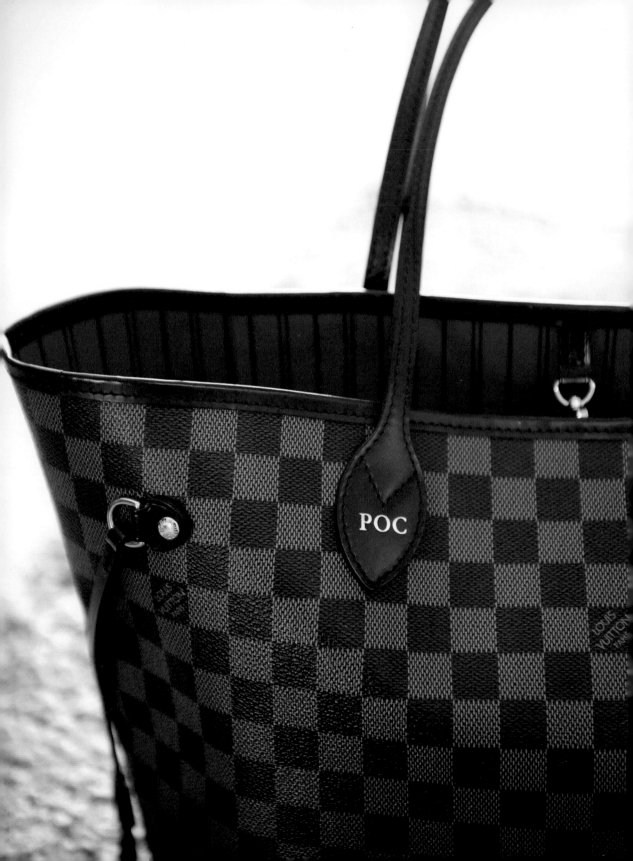

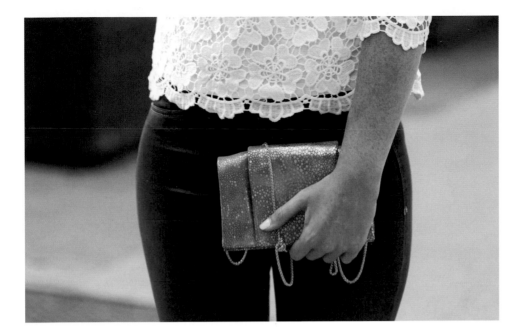

The classics that I love

- Chanel Boy bag or the flap bag

- The Celine Trapeze bag

- The Louis Vuitton Neverfull bag

I actually bought the Neverfull over a year ago. I got my initials 'POC' engraved in gold, which I love. I'm so thrilled that I bought it. Without exaggerating, I've used it most days since then. It's light, sturdy and goes with everything.

If designer bags aren't your thing, or you'd rather spend your money elsewhere, it doesn't mean you can't have a great selection of bags that look amazing. Some of my personal favourites are from high street shops like Zara and Warehouse. Both do amazing bags for every occasion.

BAGS TO HAVE IN YOUR COLLECTION

Classic tote

This is the type of bag you'll use most frequently because you really can fit everything but the kitchen sink in there. I often find Ollie's dinosaurs and cars at the bottom of mine. Black or tan would be the best buys.

Clutch

My favourite type of bag for a glam evening event. I just love clutch bags. I have them in every colour and texture from black patent to embellished with coloured crystals.

Messenger

A flat bag with a long strap that you wear across the body. Perfect for shopping, at a concert or when you're with your kids, as you have your hands free.

Wristlet

A clutch-shaped bag that comes with an attached leather or bracelet-looking strap.

Shoulder bag

A small to medium sized bag with a long leather strap or chain attached, worn on your shoulder.

Duffel bag

A large bag usually used for travel or sports.

TIPS ON HOW TO CARE
FOR YOUR HANDBAGS

Take your empty bag outside, turn it upside-down and gently shake it to remove any debris/dust. Or in my case, broken pieces of Lego belonging to my son!

- Clean the interior of your bag by gently pulling it inside out and using a lint roller. If I can't pull out the lining of a handbag, I've often used the fabric brush attachment from my Hoover.

- To help keep the interior clean, never have loose make-up lying around in your bag. Keep it in a make-up bag and always put the caps on everything, including pens. I've had black eyeliners do damage before – not good!

- Clean the exterior of any leather bag with alcohol-free baby wipes.

- If your leather bag is stained, take it to a leather expert so they can clean it professionally.

- If you've spent a lot of money on a handbag that doesn't have studs on the bottom, it may be worth considering having some put on by a leather specialist. This will protect your bag from getting scratched when you place it on the floor.

- Store your handbag in the bag it came with. If there's no bag with it you could use a pillowcase.

- When storing your bags, don't squash them tightly into boxes – they will lose their shape. Ideally store them upright in a little cubbyhole or on a shelf.

WHAT'S IN MY BAG

I love seeing what's in other people's handbags and judging by my gal pals so do we all! I think we're just nosey and find it interesting. So, today, I emptied out the contents of my Neverfull and here what was (truthfully!) inside:

- Make-up – too many lip-glosses, my Pippa palette, a brush, lipstick, mascara, concealer
- Coco Chanel perfume
- Back combing brush
- Hairspray
- Chewing gum
- Hair bobbins
- Wallet
- Loose receipts
- Raisins (for Ollie)
- Sweets (definitely mine!)
- Loose change
- Keys
- Diary
- Pens
- Tissues
- Handcream
- Deodorant
- Notebook
- Sunglasses x 2!

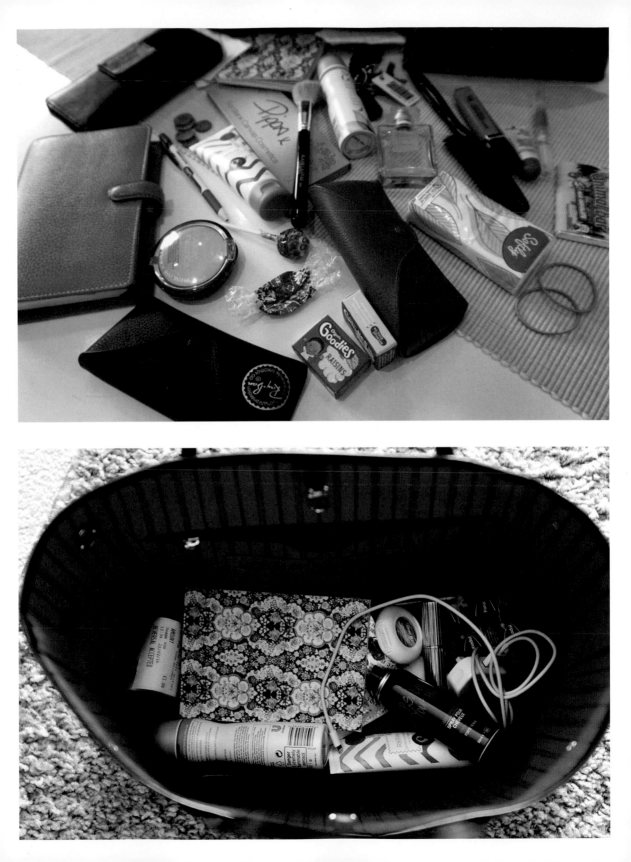

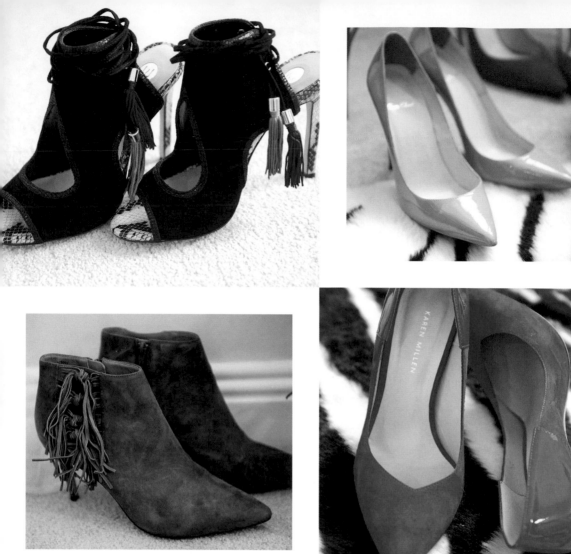

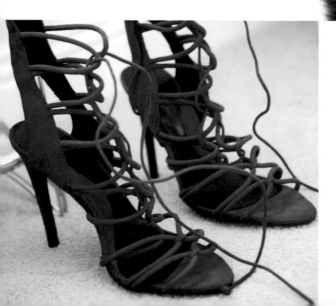

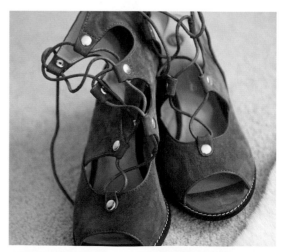

SHOES

I love shoes as much as I do handbags, probably a little more actually. So much so that, as I mentioned earlier, I got my husband to make me a shoe wall as I couldn't even walk into our spare room anymore without falling over them. Plus, I wanted to make room for baby number two! More about my shoe wall and storage later in the book.

Similar to bags, shoes will always fit regardless of losing or putting on weight. Mind you, if you're pregnant with swollen ankles, the high heels may need to be put away for a while. (Speaking of pregnancy, I definitely can't wear heels as high as I could before giving birth. Well, I do, obviously, I'm a shoe fanatic, but they're definitely not as comfy since having babies! I'm not sure what that's about.)

A few things to consider before purchasing shoes:

- Know your size. My own feet have shrunk over the years. I went from a size seven to a six. This is quite common, so it's a good idea to get measured again if you're unsure.

- Always try on both shoes in the shop, especially if you have one foot a little bigger than the other, which most of us do.

- Before you leave the shop, make sure you're getting one right and left shoe. This has happened to me on a few occasions; I've gotten home to discover I've two left feet by mistake!

- Wear your new shoes at home on the carpet to make sure you're entirely happy with them before you venture out. Just in case you need to return them.

- If shoes do feel a little tight, remember that suede and leather will stretch naturally with wear. Otherwise, you can have any shoe stretched by taking them to a cobblers.

- For shoes that are pinching you slightly, try rubbing a small bit of Vaseline on the inside to help soften the leather.

- During my ten years as a model, I walked in hundreds of fashion shows. A trick that always worked for us to avoid slipping in high heels was simply to spray hairspray onto the soles of your heels. It really works!

- There are dozens of different shoe styles and heel types. Platforms are in fashion one season and it's back to kitten heels the next. I say, just buy and wear what suits you and what you love, because shoe styles really do change so frequently.

- If you're spending a lot of money on a pair of shoes or boots that you don't want to go out of fashion, just invest wisely by opting for a simple style like flat leather black boots or a nude patent court shoe. These are safe styles that you won't tire of.

- Also, something to bear in mind is that shoes with a low-cut vamp (see page 31) instantly elongate and slenderize your leg when you're wearing skirts, shorts and dresses.

- A heel – think two and a half inches and above – lifts the body and makes clothes fall better, which gives a slimmer appearance. Look for pumps with slightly pointed toes and thin heels, as opposed to square toes, super-chunky styles or thick ankle straps, all of which can give the appearance of a shorter, stockier leg.

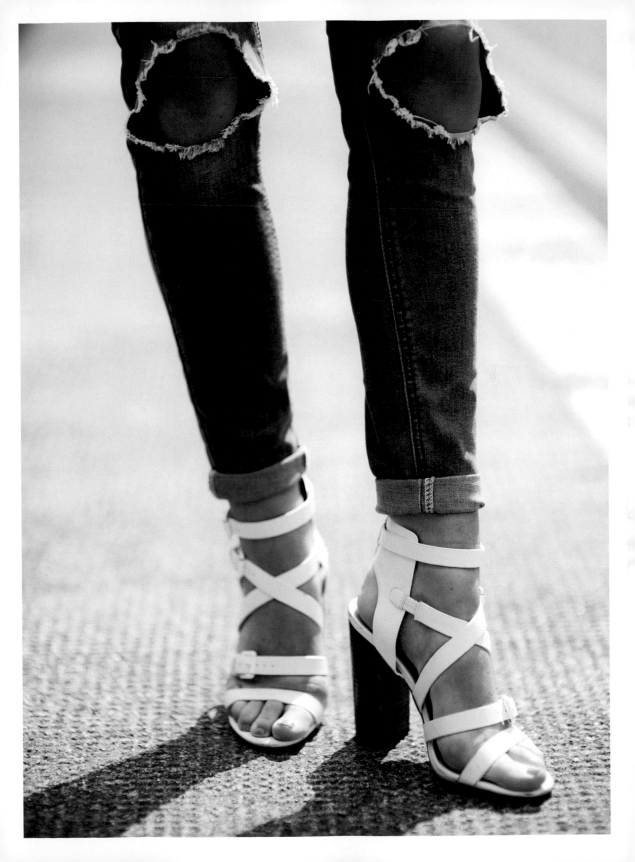

SCARVES

Scarves can take almost any outfit up a notch. They are a staple in everyone's wardrobe and they're definitely not only for the colder weather. They are probably one of my favourite accessories, whether I'm wearing a thick and cosy one on a winter's day, or a light and flowery one on a warmer spring day.

My favourite scarves are ones I've inherited from my mum, which include a large square Burberry blanket scarf that I love to wrap myself up in on chilly days. This, with a pop of red lipstick, is a gorgeous look in itself. Large square scarves can be bought in all the high street stores now, too. Zara, especially, has them at really reasonable prices.

The other scarf I have that belonged to my mum (which actually came from my granny, Dodo) is an old yellow Louis Vuitton silk and cashmere scarf. Something like this is so timeless and will never go out of fashion. So, maybe go looking through your granny's or mother's collection before hitting the shops or markets; you'd be surprised what's in fashion again or what never went out of fashion.

The possibilities for styling scarves are endless. You can opt for a big, drapey blanket scarf over a wool coat or leather jacket, or you can style up your favourite blazer with a small silk necktie to add instant glam and sophistication.

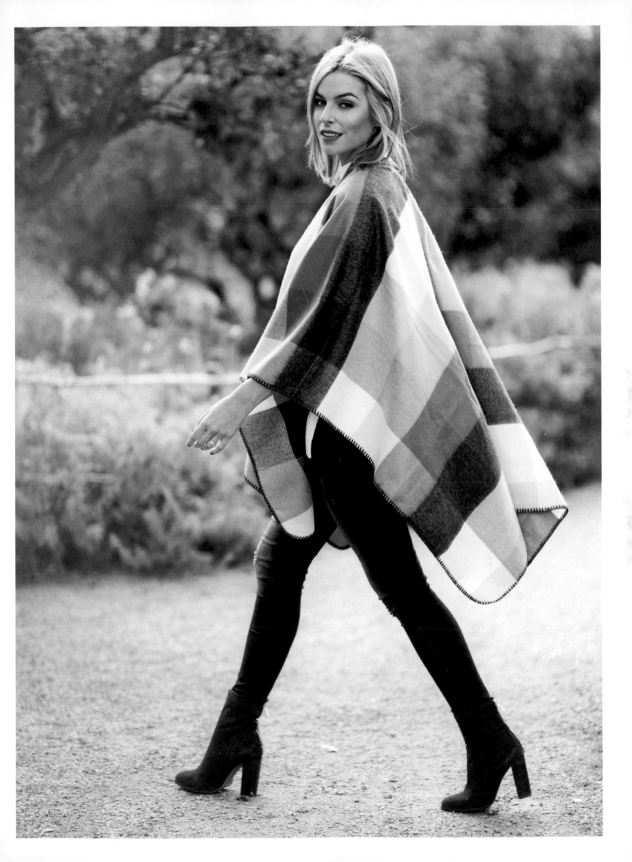

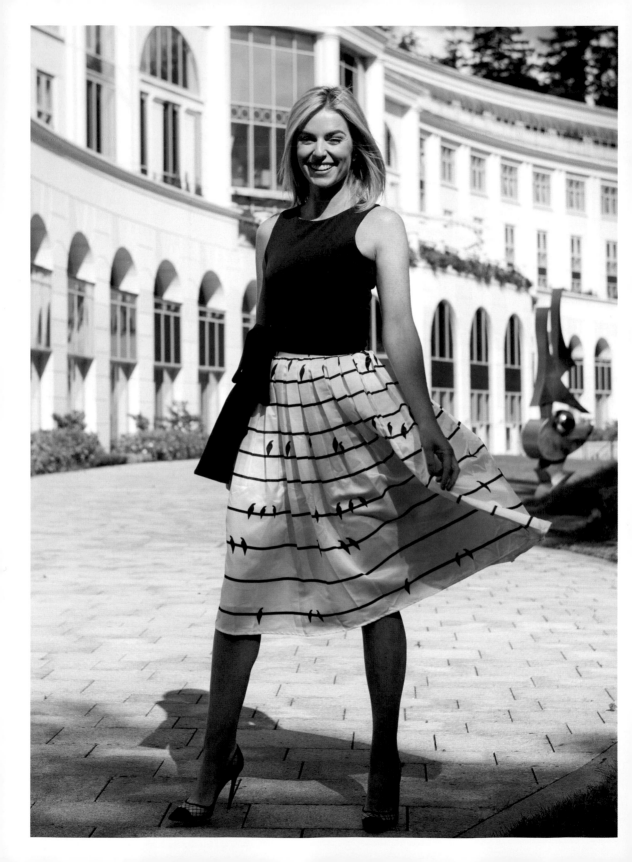

CHAPTER THREE

DRESSING FOR OCCASIONS

There are times in all our lives when what you wear is really important. Whether it's a job interview, a first date or a glamorous night out, how you look creates that vital first impression.

If you're like me, then these kind of special occasions can sometimes be a bit nerve-racking – especially if it's a first date! Many people often worry about what to wear to a wedding. Full-length dress or something less formal? Short skirt or knee-length and floaty? And what about accessories and, the item that seems to send everyone into a cold sweat, a hat? The questions are endless but don't worry as I address some of them here.

Whatever the event, it's vital you feel good about what you're wearing. You'll then feel more confident and relaxed, which will show in your body language and help to create a dazzling look for any occasion.

DRESSING FOR AN INTERVIEW

If I was interviewing for any job, the first thing I'd look for is someone who is presentable and groomed. By groomed, I mean hair blow-dried nicely, tied back or styled neatly, and nails bare or nicely painted – no chips!

Clothes should look neat, tidy and fresh. Shoes buffed. Pops of bright colour are great as it sends messages of enthusiasm and energy. They shouldn't be overpowering, though.

You also need to think carefully about whether your outfit is suitable for the role you're going for. It's probably best not to go to a teacher's interview in a mini skirt and bare legs, no matter how hot your legs are!

Whatever you're going for, you want to come across as confident and capable. If in doubt about what to wear, always go for something more formal. I go by that for any occasion I'm unsure of. It's much better to be overdressed than underdressed. Make sure, also, that you're comfortable and confident in what you're wearing – the last thing you want is a button popping off your shirt if it's a little tight.

If you're interviewing for a job at a solicitors, for instance, you could go for a tailored suit. You can still be the fashionista by teaming it with killer patent heels and a great bag. This just oozes confidence and sophistication. You also can't go wrong with a bright blouse, tailored trousers and a smart coat simply sitting on your shoulders, which you can slip off once you sit down.

✳ **TIP** *For make-up, I suggest keeping it clean and simple. Soft brown eyeshadows and nude lips. Nothing crazy. No black eye make-up or overly obvious false lashes!*

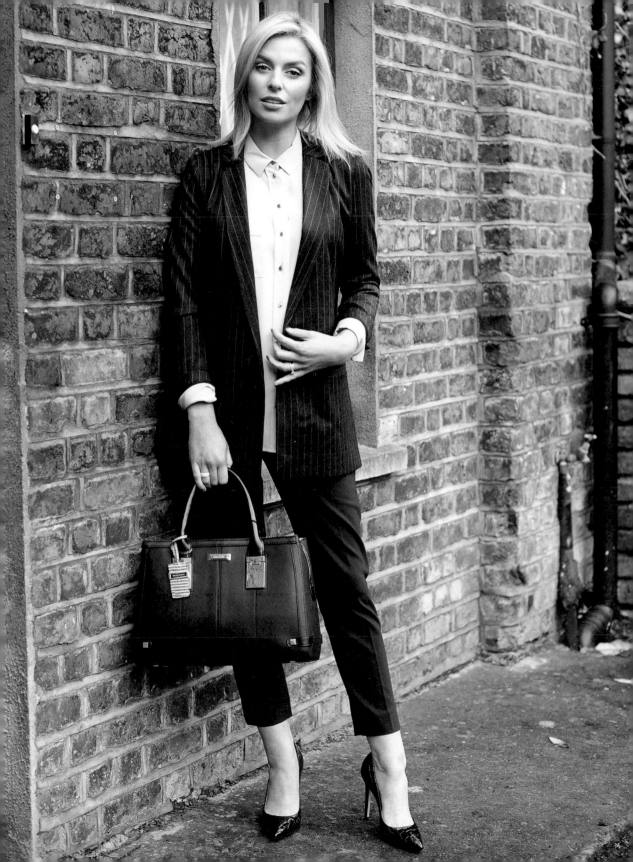

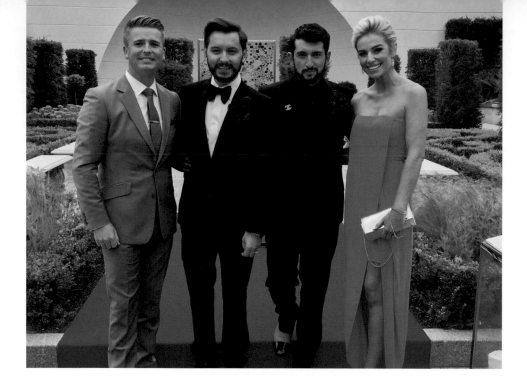

DRESSING FOR A WEDDING
OR FORMAL OCCASION

When it comes to dressing for a wedding, first things first, what's the dress code? If it isn't clearly stated on the invite, such as 'black tie', then you should just judge by the couple and the venue. Is the venue in a five-star hotel? Is the bride likely to be very glam? If yes, then go for something on the more formal side, like a fitted knee-length or below-the-knee dress. If the wedding you're attending is in a more casual location, I would still wear a dress but maybe not so formal.

Black tie

Black tie means this is formal, so ladies should ideally wear a full-length dress. It doesn't have to be black, you can go for any colour. Black tie also means the men should wear a black tuxedo with a black dickie bow or black tie.

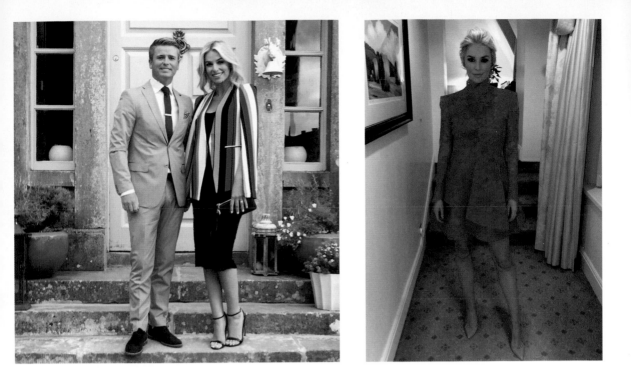

Glamorous

This is what we chose to go on our wedding invites, back in June 2011. I didn't want men to feel too formal in black, especially as it was a June wedding, so I figured glamorous was better. In other words, the ladies were free to wear short or long, as long as they felt glam! Men should wear a suit and tie.

Beach wedding

For this, a floaty knee-length dress or maxi dress is perfect. You don't necessarily have to wear heels, flats are equally appropriate. Men can wear light linen trousers and a short-sleeved shirt.

Semi-formal

I would wear a cocktail dress for this or perhaps a killer black jumpsuit accessorized with amazing statement earrings. Again, a suit and tie for the men.

WEDDING GUEST TIPS

■ Call me old-fashioned but a lady should never wear white to a wedding; it's just rude. It's the bride's day to shine.

■ Don't go too sexy. It's the bride's day, so I would never go for anything too booby or outrageous.

■ If it's winter and you're going to be in a church, make sure you have a warm coat to wear during the ceremony. In summer, bring along a wrap or pashmina to go over your shoulders in the church.

If you want to wear a hat absolutely go for it, just nothing that's going to take anyone's eye out. Wear the hat – don't let it wear you.

■ If you're the mother of one of the happy couple, then you might see this as your chance to splash out on a fabulous hat. Social convention used to dicate that the mother of the groom wear a hat smaller than the mother of the bride, so the guests would never outshine their hosts. Conventions change and, of course, vary from wedding to wedding, so if in any doubt just talk to the respective families. And if you and your groom are hosting the wedding, then the two mums could opt for equally grand creations.

■ If you don't want to wear a hat, you could still make a statement by putting a decorative clip in your hair. You can buy fantastic ones adorned with jewellery, soft feathers or with colourful flowers attached.

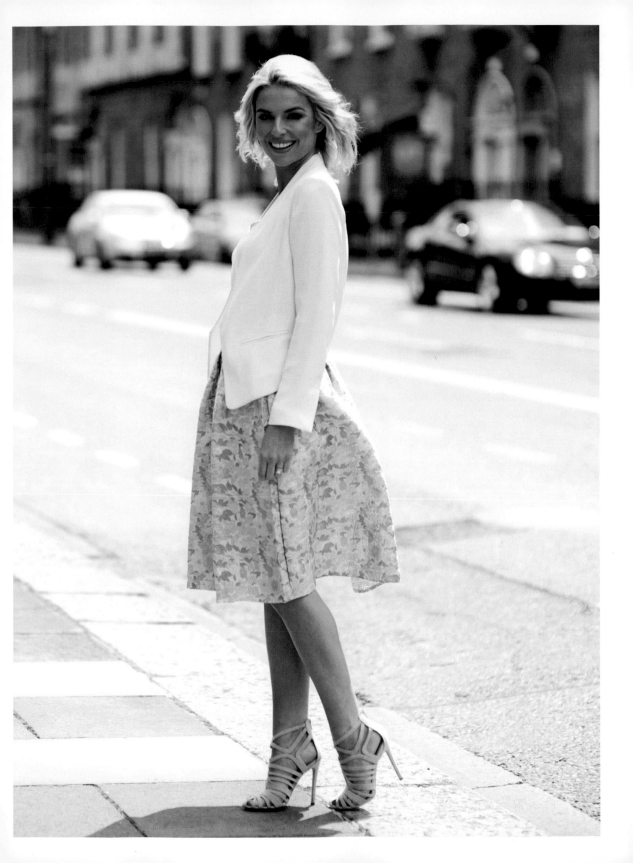

DRESSING FOR A FIRST DATE

My first date with my husband sounds so cheesy and clichéd now but it was on Valentine's night in 2008. Not only is it nerve-racking enough going on your first dinner date to a fancy restaurant, but to do it on Valentine's? Awkward much!! Saying that, eight years later we're still together and in love. I obviously nailed the outfit that night!

Dinner date

For my first dinner date with my husband, I remember wearing a short purple satin dress and high heels. It's important you're comfortable, so when choosing your outfit make sure you can sit comfortably and you feel confident in what you're wearing.

For instance, don't wear a low cut dress if you feel the urge to keep adjusting yourself and don't wear anything that you could potentially slip out of. (Not what we want on the first date!)

Make sure you're not wearing anything that's too tight. You want to eat and actually enjoy the food with your date! If in doubt, black is always a good choice. A simple black dress accessorized to your liking will take you anywhere.

Make sure you have eaten something during the day of your dinner date, otherwise you'll be tipsy before the meal even arrives!

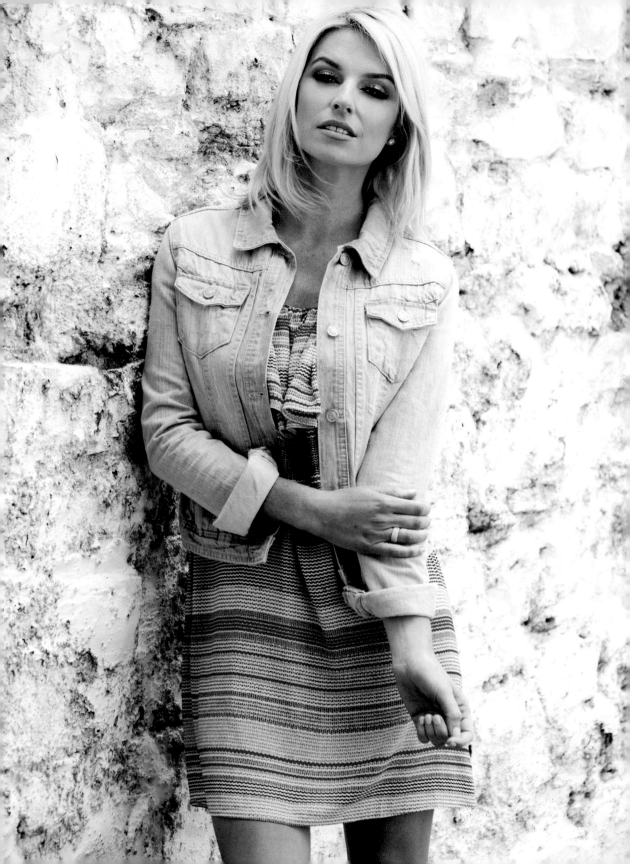

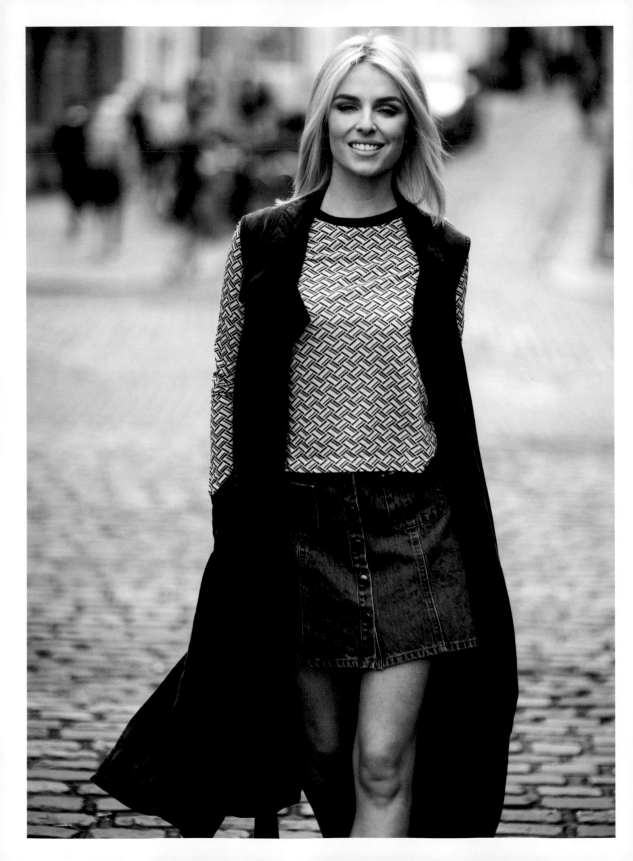

Coffee date

This is the type of date I'd recommend most to my friends. Especially if you haven't met your date before, it's going to be the most casual and easy way to meet. Plus, you don't have to go to the expense of getting an outfit or having your hair and make-up done as you might for a dinner date. Save that for when you know you like each other!

For a coffee date, you might be meeting on your work lunch break so you'll be wearing whatever you wear to work, which is fine. Otherwise, I'd go for something really simple like my favourite jeans, shirt and trainers or a short casual daytime skirt with flats, and a casual top teamed with a duster coat or oversized knit.

Cinema date

Similar to your coffee date, wear something cool and casual. There's definitely no need for your high heels on this occasion. At most, I'd wear my wedge runners with jeans and a pretty top. Don't forget to have them loose enough so you can enjoy all the cinema treats.

Bar date

If you're meeting your date in a bar for a few casual drinks, I'd go for the less-is-more 'I'm such a cool chick' look. I'm thinking leather trousers, a good quality basic tee tucked into one side. Some really cool bangles stacked up, or a beautiful pair of earrings, with my favourite pair of sexy shoes. Hair tousled and undone-looking (obviously it's just been done to look undone!). Often these dates are overthought when, really, less is certainly more and shows a laid-back, I'm-not-trying-hard attitude!

DRESSING FOR THE RACES

Horse racing is a really popular sporting and social event. However, deciding what to wear to the races can leave most of us a little stuck. The dresses in our wardrobe are either too short or impractically long. So, what should you go for?

For a dress or skirt, I suggest a hem length that is midi or just to the knee – this is most appropriate for daytime wear. An A-line shape is always flattering as it nips you in at the waist. It's a great look on all ages too. I absolutely love something like a full midi skirt with a fine knit tucked in.

Depending on the time of year, it's important to dress appropriately for the weather. Racecourses can be very cold (I'm thinking of Ireland here) so be sure you're warm enough. If it's winter, I'd plan my outfit around a beautiful coat and let that be your focal point.

Gone are the days that every item of your outfit has to be matching, complete with a frilly Mary Poppins-like umbrella!

Think outside the box and let your personality shine. Don't be afraid to clash your prints or colours – just don't go too overboard. You might like to choose a theme for your outfit like monochrome – I adore black and white as it's classy, elegant and appropriate for any time of year.

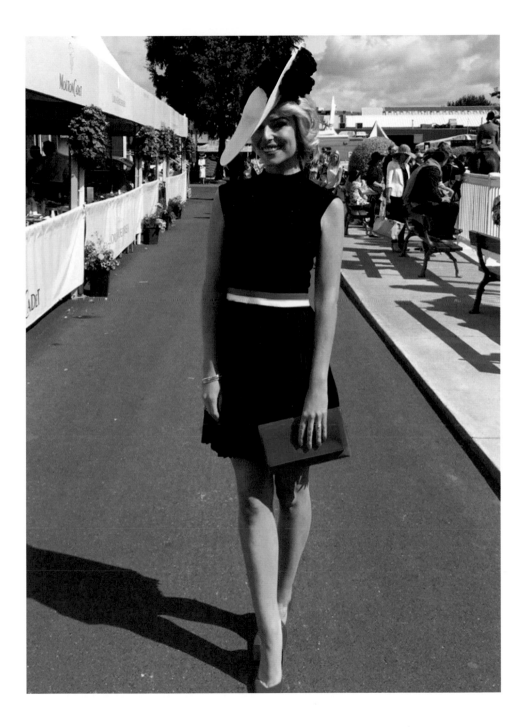

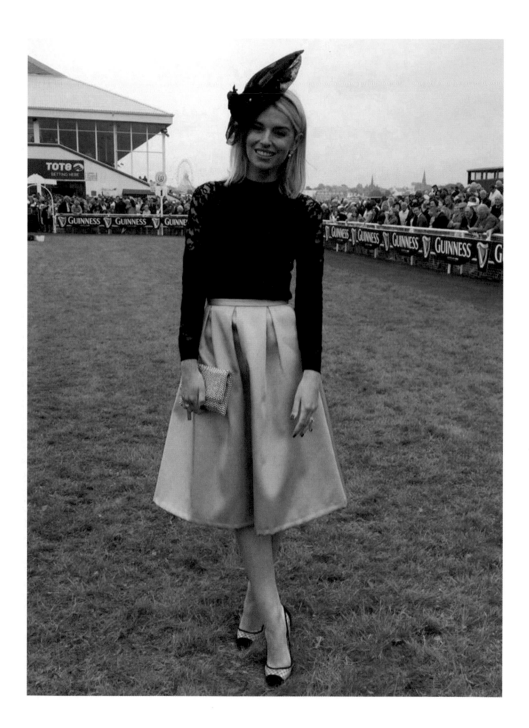

It's a great occasion to wear an amazing hat and really go all out. If you're going to do so, it's a good idea to have your hair professionally styled and your hat placed securely on with the help of your hairdresser to make sure it's comfortable and stays in place. (It's often quite windy standing on the side of a racecourse!)

Accessorizing your outfit is another brilliant way to stand out at the races. So, for instance, you could wear a plain black dress with orange heels and a floral print clutch bag. It's the combination of the whole look that'll get you noticed for all the right reasons.

Some points to keep in mind:

- If you want to look elegant and feel comfortable all day, stay away from very short skirts and teeny-weeny dresses with lots of skin on show.

- Choose shoes that are comfortable and not too high – it can be a long day at the races.

- If wearing tights, bring a spare pair, just in case!

- If you wear fake tan, don't go overboard with it. Everything shows up in the daylight and you don't want to look too mucky or orange.

- Be confident and comfortable-looking. I've judged so many ladies' days over the years and this kind of thing is what I look for above anything. To me there's nothing more stylish than a confident-looking woman.

DRESSING FOR A CASUAL BUT CHIC EVENT

We all know how hard it can be to nail looking casual but cool at the same time. You don't want to look like you're trying too hard but you still want your outfit to work well and look like you've made an effort, if only just a bit!

So what exactly is 'casual chic'? It's all about being comfortable but still on trend. Style is not sacrificed for comfort (or vice versa) when it comes to casual chic dressing, and that's why it's my favourite everyday style.

If you're going to a friend's birthday brunch, for example, you don't want to look too done up, as if you're going out at nighttime. The key is to keep everything simple and elegant. Let your accessories and shoes elevate your look.

Start with your staple wardrobe pieces. I think you can never go wrong with a simple pair of skinny jeans and a plain tee. Inject a pop of colour to your look with your shoes and add a statement necklace for some extra glamour. I'd throw on a leather biker jacket to give the outfit some edge or a simple blazer for the ultimate chic look.

I think Olivia Palermo has casual chic dressing down to a T. She makes everything look so effortless but still very fashionable and put together. I always look to her and other street style bloggers for inspiration.

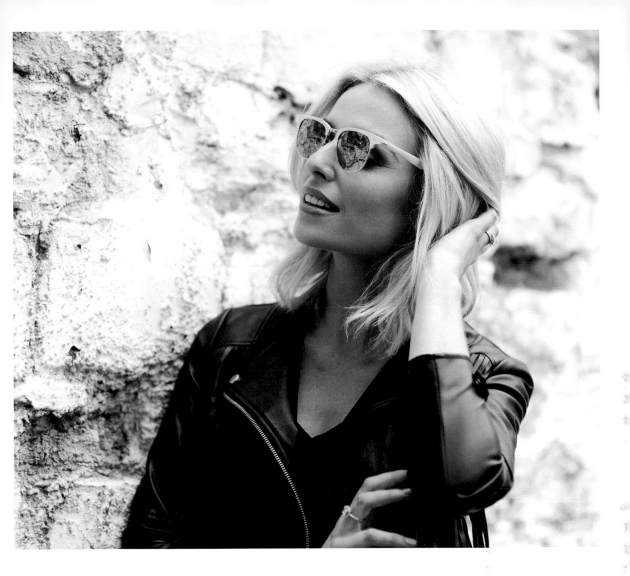

You want to feel like yourself in what you're wearing, so don't worry about going for an old favourite in your wardrobe if it's comfortable and you know it suits you. Rotate your basics and there's no shame in wearing something more than two or three times – even Olivia recycles her key staple pieces. Sometimes, a lot of us forget that everything in our wardrobe can be styled differently each time we wear it. And the addition of some statement jewellery and accessories can be major style game-changers, changing your entire look completely.

Be soft. Do not let the world make you hard. Do not let pain make you hate. Do not let the bitterness steal your sweetness. Take pride that even though the rest of the world may disagree, you still believe it to be a beautiful place.

Iain S. Thomas

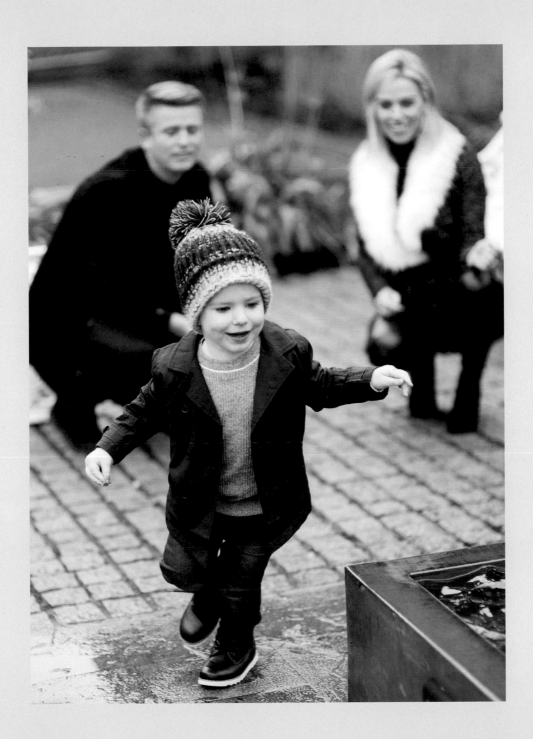

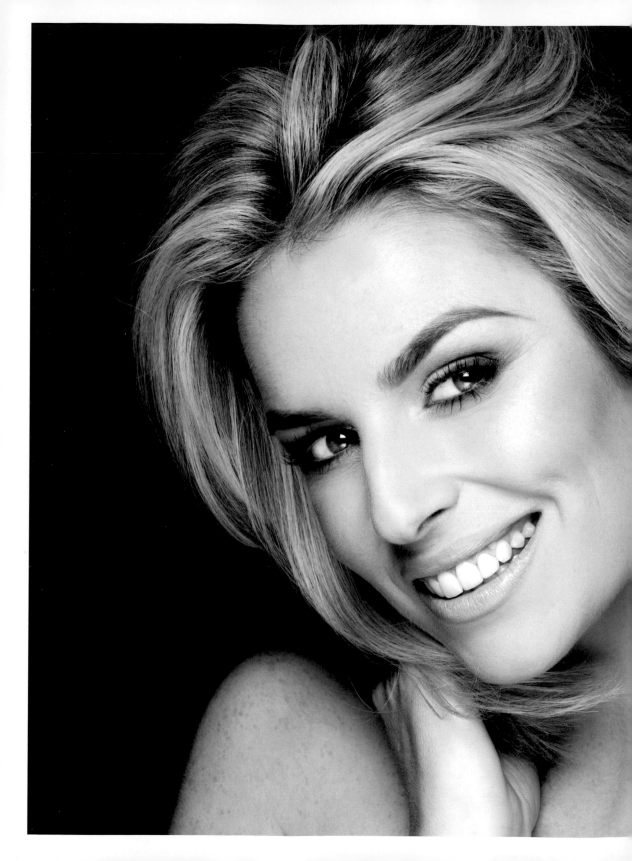

PART TWO: BEAUTY

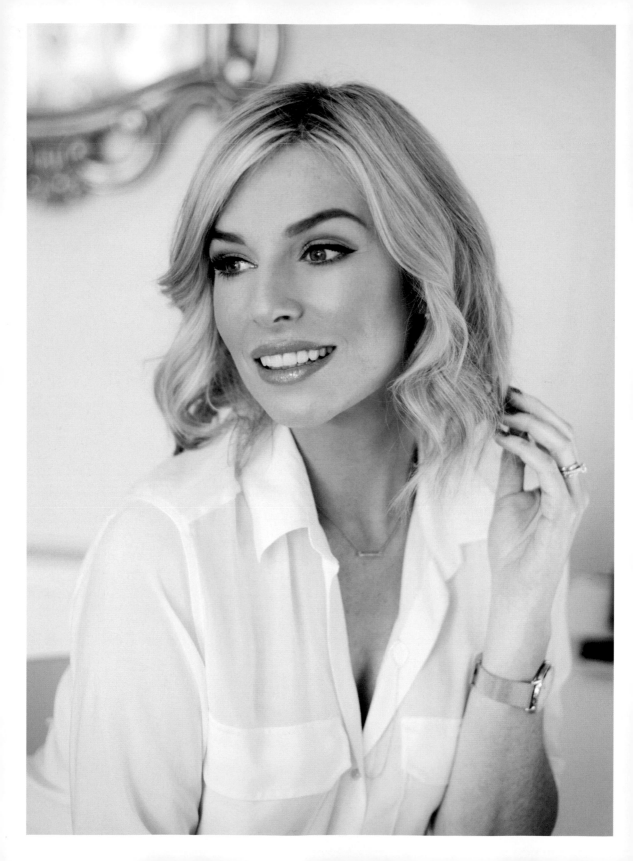

CHAPTER FOUR

FEELING BEAUTIFUL

Feeling beautiful and looking your best is important to so many of us. My feeling is that no matter who you are, when you look awful, you feel awful – and who wants to feel like that?

On the odd occasion that I make absolutely no effort, I never have a good day, because I just don't feel good about myself. I hate having unwashed hair and a pasty white face. So, even if it's just putting on some tinted moisturizer and a coloured lipgloss – the difference it makes in how I feel is unbelievable.

It's not about impressing others. For me it's beside the point who will see me, it's about making a little bit of effort to feel good about myself. (Saying that, on days when simply getting out the door with your child is a major triumph, I do get that putting on a bit of lippy can move down the to-do list.) The same applies to clothes. If I ever feel slobby or I'm wearing something I don't particularly feel good in, I don't have a good day. So, I simply don't do that to myself.

The power of make-up really is remarkable. My mum used to say. 'Once I have my face on, I'm ready for anything' – and it's so true. Yes, it's good to embrace your natural beauty and have no make-up days, and I think it's important not to feel the need for it all the time … But, on the other hand, isn't it amazing what make-up can do for us as women? There's nothing more satisfying than buying a new lipstick – cheap therapy if you ask me!!

Growing up, I went through many awkward stages of dodgy hair and make-up. I had black hair, red hair, orange hair (that was supposed to be blonde!) along with white make-up that made me look like a scary goth, and blue shimmery eyeshadow brought up to my eyebrows. Speaking of eyebrows, mine were so over-plucked and over-arched I resembled a cartoon character!

Then, there was my obsession with fake tan. Why didn't anybody tell me 'less is more'? Actually, I'm sure my poor mum went blue in the face telling me, but as a teen and twenty-something I probably thought, what does she know, so I did it anyway!

As I've gone from my mid twenties to thirties I've realized that 'less is more' is definitely the way to go. Although, the silly mistakes we make as we grow up help us to find our individual style and how to make the best of ourselves.

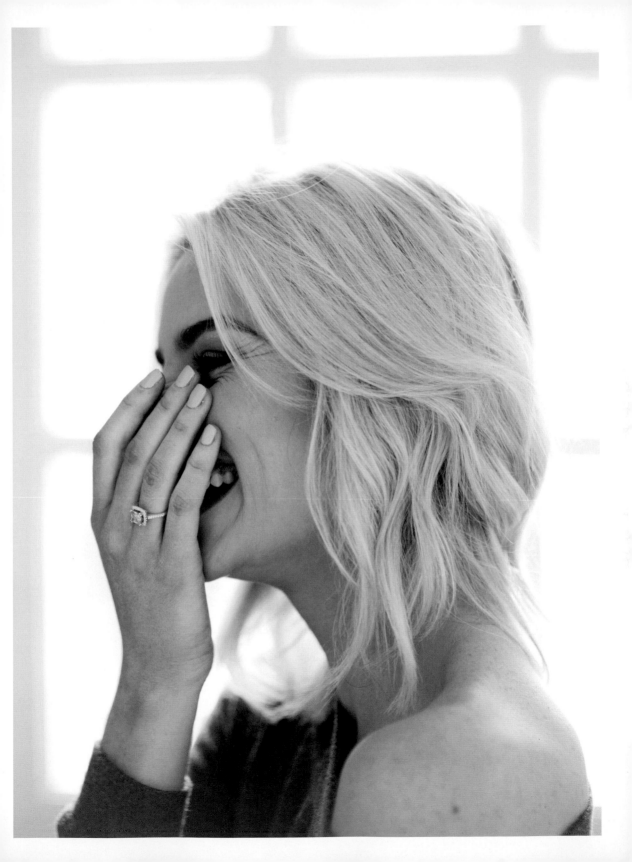

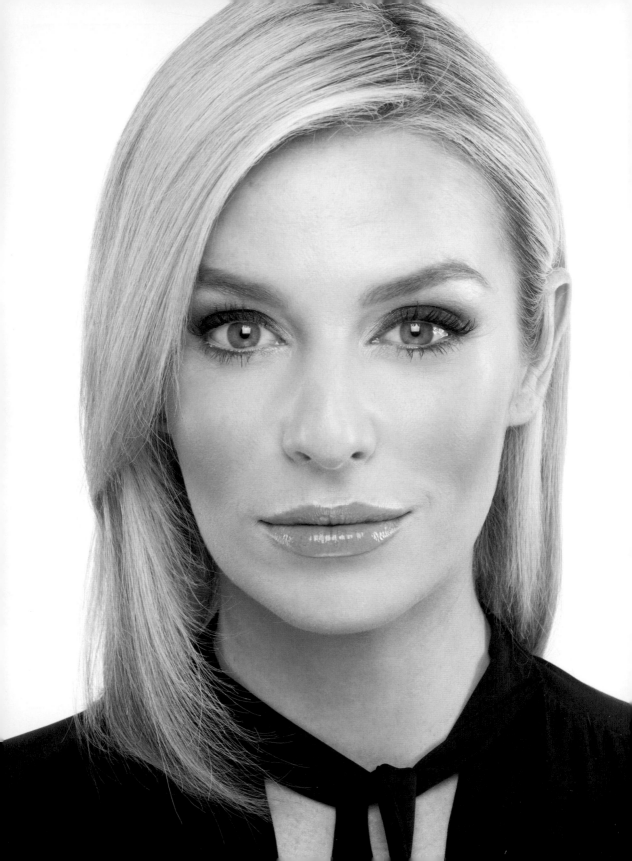

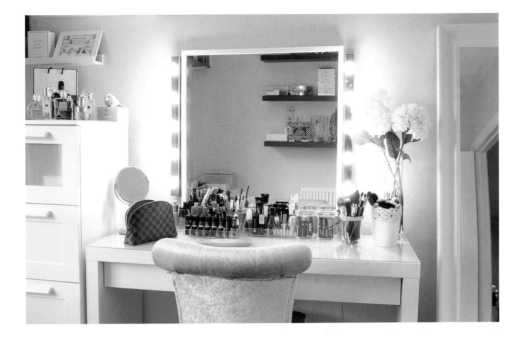

I still absolutely love make-up, now more than ever actually, as I really know what suits me. I'm not a make-up artist or qualified skin specialist, but I have lots of tips and knowledge to help other busy, everyday women. I'm not into full-on make-up and really false-looking lashes. When it comes to spending time on make-up application, I'm actually bordering on lazy. For everyday wear, I want everything done quickly and easily.

Sure, I spend longer getting ready for a night out or work event. And when I have the time, I'll close the door in my make-up room, turn on some music and have a bit of 'me time'. I really enjoy it and there's no better feeling than getting made-up. In this book, I'll be sharing with you some of these more glamorous make-up looks but I'm just as excited to share my quick guides on how to get ready in minutes, and with a toddler hanging from your leg!

A GOOD SKINCARE ROUTINE

Before I get into make-up, I'm going to focus on skincare and my own routines. I'm really into caring for my skin now, and buying the right skincare products and creams will sometimes take priority over make-up, purely because it's a better investment in the long run. Well cared for skin will age less and look better with make-up, and really clean skin will absorb more moisture.

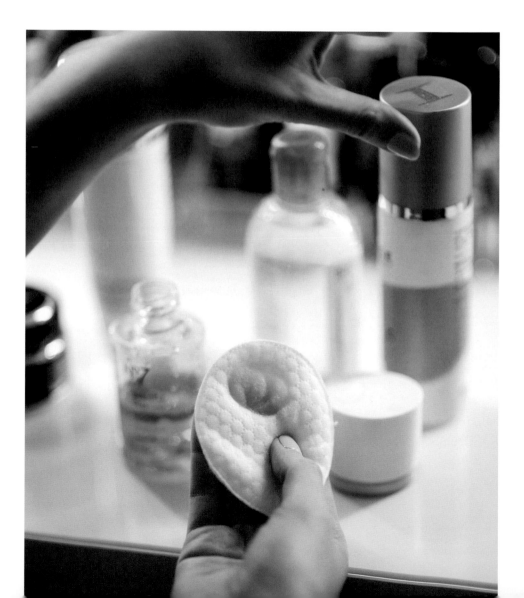

As a teenager, I had terrible skin. I mean really bad – I was covered in spots with 'bullet holes', as my brother Cian would refer to them, all over my face. Today, I still have a couple of scars from back then. I never took acne medication, I just weathered the storm and piled on the concealer (not ideal!). I wish I had known then what I know now, which is how to cleanse my face correctly and the importance of knowing my skin type.

Back then, I also wish I had known that face wipes weren't doing me any favours. They only remove the top layer of what's on your face, and don't give your skin a deep cleanse in order to remove all the dirt and grime. My rules now for face wipes are that you should only resort to them on certain occasions:

1 If you've had too many drinks after a night out, using a face wipe is definitely better than doing nothing.

2 When you're travelling on a long flight or journey.

3 When you're at a festival!

I added a fourth exception only this week, though – my poor sister Susanna had to rush to hospital with her son by ambulance after an accident. I quickly packed an overnight bag for them. The next day, after everything was okay, she phoned me laughing, saying, 'Remind me not to ask you to pack anything in a hurry – there wasn't even a facewipe in the bag.' Silly me!

So, other than those four situations, forget about them!

 TIP *An alternative for face wipes: micellar water! This has become so popular over the last year. It's a cleansing water that literally takes everything off, including eye make-up. Perfect for lazy days! I like the micellar water from* **Bioderma** *or* **Garnier.**

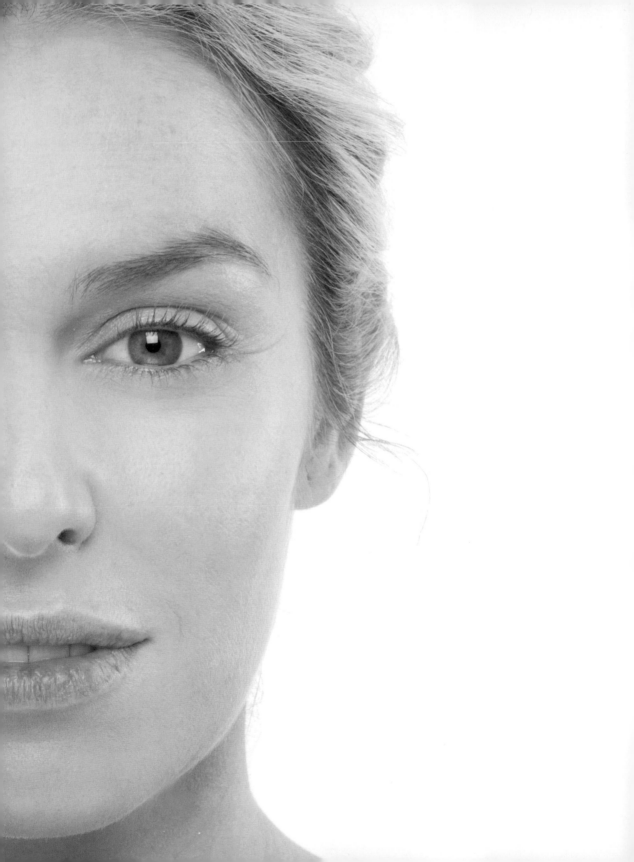

KNOWING YOUR SKIN TYPE

So, what is your skin type? Lots of people actually have no idea what skin type they are because they don't examine their faces bare, without any kind of make-up or skincare products. Take a good look at your skin, preferably in natural light and before applying any make-up (the morning is usually best).

Dry skin

Dry skin occurs when the dermis (the layer of skin that contains blood capillaries, hair follicles and other structures) does not secrete enough oil, or sebum. As a result, your skin might feel tight and be prone to flake, and you may have a dull complexion. In more extreme cases, dry skin lacks elasticity and can be extremely sensitive to the sun, wind and cold temperatures. A rich protective moisturizer will help dry skin, as will gentle cleansing – go for liquid foundations or hydrating powder foundations that deliver a little moisture to the skin.

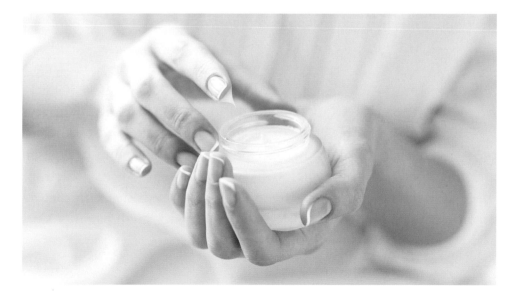

Oily skin

Oily skin is shiny skin, especially in the T-zone (from the forehead, down the nose to the chin). You may have enlarged pores and be prone to blackheads and breakouts due to overproduction by the sebaceous (oil-producing) glands. It's vital to thoroughly clean the skin on a regular basis with a gentle, soap-free cleanser, and use an oil-free or powder foundation. Mineral make-up, which is free from additives and chemicals, often works well on oily skin because its particles absorb moisture.

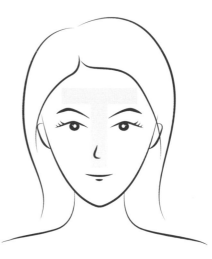

The good thing about oily skin is that it ages better than dry skin (lucky devils) because the oils keep the skin plump, allowing fewer wrinkles to form. Many young women have oily skin but, as they age, they may find their skin becomes more dry.

Sensitive skin

Sensitive skin tends to be thin and delicate with fine pores. It is easily irritated by the sun. Certain cosmetic products can cause red or angry-looking skin. It can be itchy, or blotchy in places. Choose skincare products that cater for sensitive skin, preferably labelled hypoallergenic and fragrance-free as they're less likely to cause an adverse reaction. Mineral make-up can also be a good choice for sensitive skin. Before putting anything on your face, test products on a small patch of skin and wait for 24 hours to see if any irritation occurs.

Combination skin

Most women have combination skin, which means you may have a slightly oily T-zone (around the nose and cheeks) and drier cheeks with dry patchy spots here and there. You may also have larger pores on your cheeks and possibly your forehead. This skin type generally has medium pores, a smooth and even texture, good circulation and a healthy colour. You may need to treat each area of your face differently, both in your skincare routine and when applying foundation, using oil-free make-up in oily areas and vice versa.

Normal skin

Normal skin shows neither oil nor flaking skin. It should feel supple and smooth. If you have it, consider yourself lucky! All sorts of skincare products and foundations will work well on your skin.

If, after looking at your skin, you're still unsure about your skin type, it's best to visit a professional, such as a dermatologist or beauty therapist, and they can advise you. Lots of salons offer this service for free, so have a look in your area.

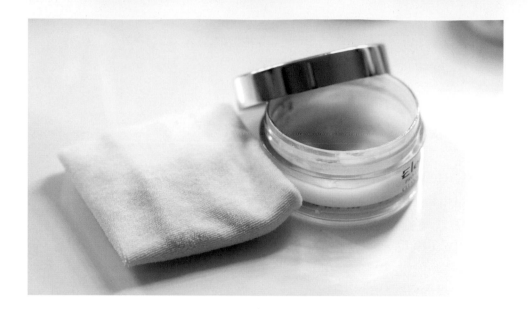

HOW TO CLEANSE YOUR FACE

There are so many different ways to cleanse your skin. You can use a facial wash, cream, oil or, my personal favourite, a balm. I love the feeling of a cleansing balm and I love how well this method removes my make-up and properly cleans my skin. I cleanse my face twice a day, in the morning and evening.

First, I remove my eye make-up using an eye make-up remover and cotton pad. I like using one that is oil-based because it quickly and effectively removes everything, even waterproof mascara. Don't use an oil-based remover if you have semi-permanent lashes. It'll destroy them. Use an oil-free one, soak some onto a cotton bud and gently cleanse your eye make-up off around your lashes.

Then, using my fingers, I gently massage a big dollop of my cleansing balm all around my face and neck – avoiding the eye area. Always massage it in using upward strokes – never drag your skin down when applying anything. We want to keep everything uplifted for as long as possible!

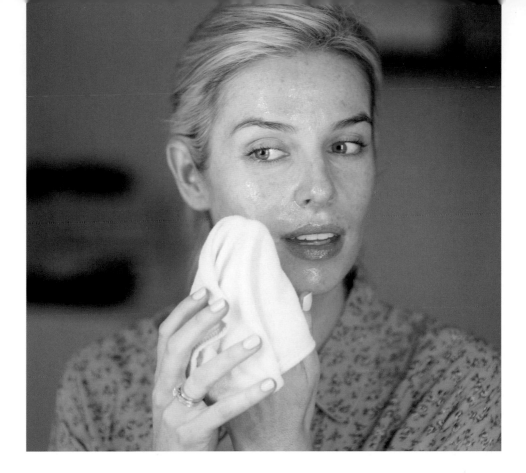

To remove the cleansing balm, I always always use a muslin cloth or face cloth. In some situations I've had to use a cotton pad to remove the balm or just washed it off with water but this won't remove all the make-up and dead skin cells.

I have two balms that I adore, they are **Elemis Pro-Collagen Cleansing Balm** and **Emma Hardie Moringa Cleansing Balm** – both are fantastic in my opinion but, really, it's the method that's important, not so much the product.

I always recommend double cleansing – so repeat the cleansing balm method twice. If you haven't tried this before, give it a go. I promise you'll never clean your face another way again!

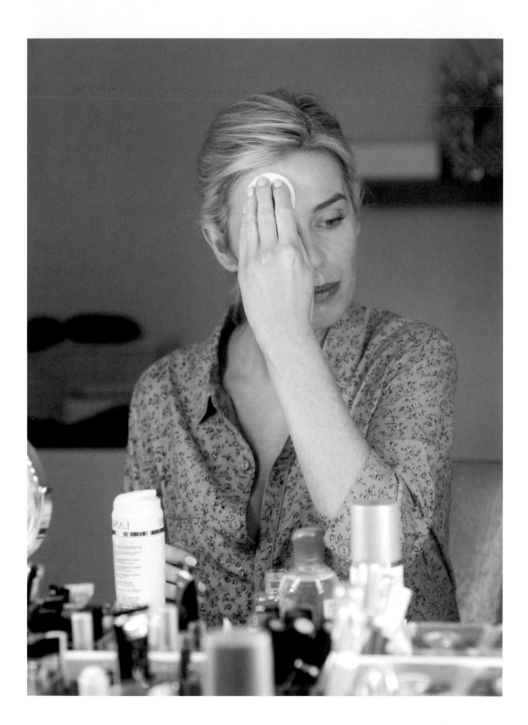

Toners

I tend to use a toner most mornings and evenings after I've cleansed. This isn't an essential step, though – I just like how it makes my skin feel. If you've cleansed your skin properly you shouldn't need to do much else before you apply your moisturizer.

I like a toner that exfoliates and brightens and I use **First Aid Beauty Facial Radiance Pads** for this.

Serums

I love serums and use them every day. I apply every morning before my moisturizer and every evening before my night cream, and they've made such a difference to my skin.

Serums provide real nourishment to the skin and are used to treat all sorts of skin issues from spots to dehydrated skin and wrinkles. Like all skincare, you need to decide exactly what's right for your skin but there's certainly a serum for everyone and all ages should be using one. I use a couple of different serums, depending on what I want them for, such as any redness or dry areas. You can also use a different one in the morning to your evening one to treat various concerns. I like **Image Skincare** in general but their **Vital C Serum** is particularly good.

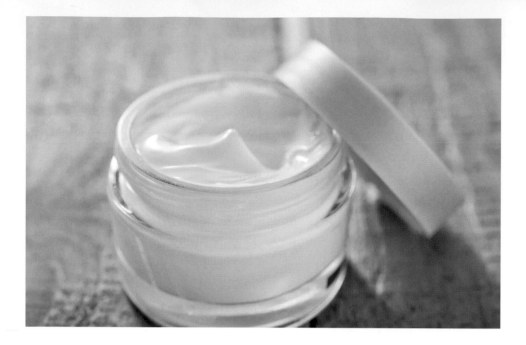

Eye creams

Yes, everybody should be using eye cream. If you're reading this now and thinking, oh, I don't have an eye cream, that's okay – just start tomorrow!

The skin around your eyes is so thin and sensitive that your regular moisturizer is too heavy for the area. So, leave it free from moisturizer and only use your eye cream here. Too much eye cream or a heavy moisturizer under the eyes can cause milia, which are those little white lumps people often experience. Be gentle when applying your eye cream. You only need a tiny, tiny amount. Apply to your ring fingers and gently pat all around your eye area.

My personal favourites are **Image Vital C**, **Image The Max** and **Dermalogica Multivitamin Power Firm**. People often ask me what product will get rid of dark circles. Truthfully? None. Unfortunately, it's usually genetic. You can just cleverly conceal them, and I'll go over this in my make-up section.

Moisturizers

Even my husband uses a moisturizer – so, thankfully, we're both on the same page in terms of knowing they're good and we need them.

For my day moisturizer, I always use one with an SPF (sun protection factor) in it – even in winter, don't underestimate the importance of an SPF. For overnight, I use a specific night cream that's usually a little heavier. You can use a night oil or serum under this, and I apply my moisturizer after my eye cream. Again, it's about what you require. Personally, I like using everything at nighttime as your skin is most absorbent then. Also, you don't need to worry about make-up sliding off if you're using an oil.

Your choice when it comes to moisturizers is endless, so it's really about personal preference and choosing what is right for your skin type. Dry, flaky skin might require a rich, protective moisturizer; oily skin an oil-free, lighter moisturizer and sensitive skin a fragrance-free moisturizer, labelled 'hypoallergenic' or 'for sensitive skin'. Cold weather and air conditioning (especially in planes) will also dry out the skin, so you may need to apply more moisturizer than usual in these conditions (along with a good lip balm).

Did you know?

A moisturizer containing an SPF can cause you to look like a ghost in a photograph. Have you ever wondered why your face is white and body is tanned? It's because the SPF is causing flashback. Obviously, don't ditch the SPF, but for a night out or an occasion where pictures are going to be taken, avoid using anything with an SPF.

Exfoliators

Exfoliation removes the top layers of dead skin cells to reveal a fresher, more radiant skin. I like to exfoliate about twice a week, after cleansing but before toning or moisturizing. You can use a liquid exfoliator – one of my favourite methods – which is very simple and quick to use. You just dab some onto a cotton pad and sweep over the face. I like an exfoliant containing glycolic as that's good for anti-ageing and treating fine lines.

You can also exfoliate using an exfoliating scrub or face mask. My favourite exfoliating mask is definitely **Glam Glows Tinglexfoliate**, rightly dubbed the 'facial in a jar'!

Another exfoliating and cleansing tool I really like (usually I'd stay clear of any gadgets but this is my exception) is the **Clarisonic Cleansing Brush**. I came across it while I was in New York about three years ago. I was only about ten weeks pregnant with Ollie and my skin was terrible. I was breaking out in spots every second day.

So, off I went to Bloomingdales in search of even more make-up and something to cover these bad boys up!! While being sold a million products at the Armani counter, my very funny and very camp sales assistant said to me, 'Girlfriend, what are you cleaning your face with?' I told him, 'Oh, you know, the usual.' To which, he replied, 'You haven't lived until you've used the Clarisonic!'

So, obviously, I then HAD to buy this little dream machine. I felt a little robbed and silly that he'd talked me into spending over a hundred dollars on this cleansing brush. But, honestly, I'm now so glad I did! The first time I used it, I was impressed. It's not a harsh brushing motion, but it felt firm enough to really clean my skin. You simply follow the 'beep alerts' that tell you when to move on to a new part of your face. It claims to remove six times more make-up than manual cleansing, and to cleanse so well that products absorb better – making skin more receptive to skincare ingredients.

The first noticeable result was the smoothness of my face. I mean, baby-skin soft. I couldn't stop touching it! The second noticeable result was the way my make-up went on. My liquid foundation felt smoother, and my make-up seemed fresher. I use it now maybe once or twice a week.

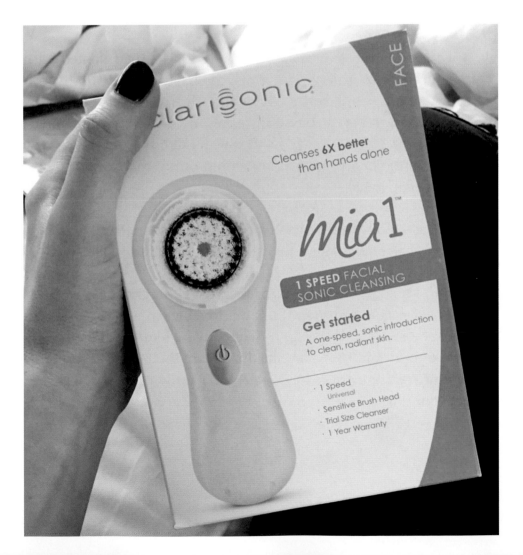

HAIR REMOVAL

Let's talk hair removal, ladies! I think it's safe to say it's not one of those tasks that we particularly enjoy, but it's a necessary one for most of us. In saying that, if you're happy with your hairy bits then by all means embrace them! I personally hate the feeling of hairy legs – I don't feel right if I have stubbly or hairy legs. To me it's like having a chipped nail – irritating and annoying.

Shaving

I've tried it all when it comes to hair removal. I experimented with shaving my legs at a very young age, probably twelve or thirteen – which was too young really as I'm sure this made my hairs grow thicker and darker. I even shaved my arms once – no, not my armpits, my actual arms! Don't ask, I've no idea why I did that! A bit like, why did I get a tattoo of a heart on the bottom of my back aged sixteen? Stupidity – that's why!

Anyway, back to my arms. Shaving them really was a bad idea. They took ages to grow back. Plus a totally hair-free arm just looked weird.

Nowadays, I tend not to use a razor to shave – I might use one under my arms every now and then if I haven't had them waxed. If using a razor, just be mindful to change it frequently – a blunt razor can easily give you a nasty cut. Use some shaving cream too. Another top tip is to use hair conditioner or shaving oil for a really close shave and to protect your skin.

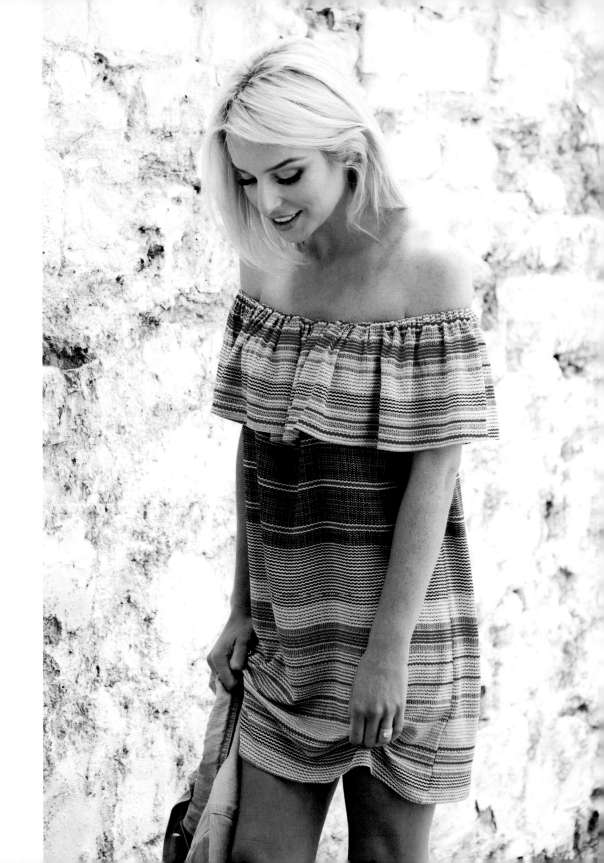

Laser hair removal

About four years ago, I tried laser hair removal. This is where highly concentrated light is beamed into the hair follicle. Pigments in the follicle absorb the light, which then damages them enough to hinder future growth. There is also IPL (intense pulsed light) hair removal, which emits light in specific wavelengths to target hair reduction.

Laser hair removal is one of the priciest ways to remove hair but it's meant to be permanent. I can't say this was the case for me – I had six or seven treatments done on my legs, bikini area and underarms, and while it reduced the hair significantly, it didn't fully remove it for good. It worked best on my underarms and I've very little hair there now.

It could be I needed more treatments for my skin and hair type, but I couldn't when I got pregnant as you can't have laser treatment when you're expecting.

The treatment itself doesn't take too long and isn't too uncomfortable – it's like a rubber band being flicked quickly and repeatedly onto your skin. It's nothing unbearable. The best results are often achieved on people with dark hair and fair skin.

Waxing

Nowadays, my preferred form of hair removal is waxing, which, thankfully, is not quite as painful as it once was! Waxing removes hair from the root and can last up to six weeks. I've found that areas I've had continuously waxed now have permanently reduced numbers of hairs.

There are two types of wax, hot and strip. A hot wax is perfect for sensitive areas like your face, underarm and bikini area. Usually an oil is applied first, to create a barrier, then hot wax is applied. This is allowed to cool, and is then pulled away from the skin in a fast movement.

Wax strips (pieces of paper with wax on them) are generally used on the legs. This is a 'cold' method of waxing, with strips applied in the direction the hair grows, smoothed over and then ripped off quickly in the opposite direction.

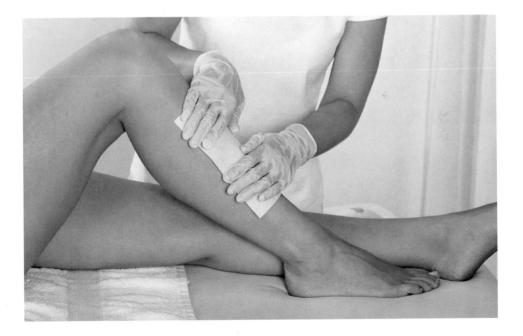

If you haven't been to a salon before for waxing but you'd like to try it, my advice is to give it a go. Don't be embarrassed – especially if you're getting your bikini area waxed for the first time. Go to a reputable salon and your therapist will be a professional. She will have seen it all before and I guarantee you she won't be the slightest bit embarrassed, so neither should you be.

Aftercare

After waxing or shaving I like to use **Waxperts** lavender oil, which soothes and softens the skin – it can be used straight after you've shaved or been waxed, which I like. The lavender oil is nice and relaxing to use before bed, too, as an all over body oil. You should also avoid using perfume or harsh deodorants for 24 hours after waxing or shaving.

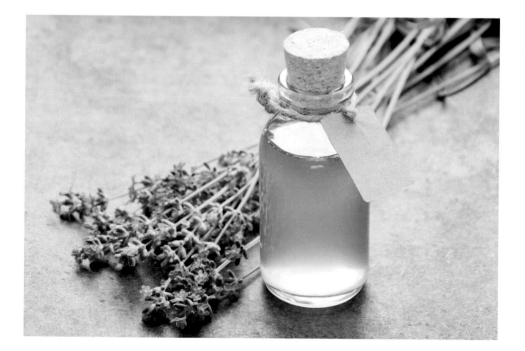

TOP BEAUTY TIPS & SECRETS

Water, water and more water...

It sounds simple, but we underestimate the importance of drinking lots of water. It's not only good for your skin, it keeps headaches at bay, boosts your energy, helps you exercise better, aids concentration and also helps with weight loss – often we confuse hunger with thirst. I typically drink 1.5 to 2 litres per day.

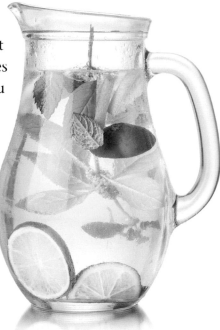

TIP *Try adding some cucumber and lemon slices to a big jug of water and leave in the fridge, or add to your water bottle when you're on the go. I love fresh mint leaves added to water too.*

Body brush

Before you get into the shower, brush your body from your feet up with a body brush (this method works best on dry skin). Use a wooden paddle with bristles; most pharmacies have these now. By massaging the skin in a circular upwards motion, these brushes help to stimulate circulation and blood flow, and remove dead skin cells. They are ideal for dry skin, which needs regular exfoliation. They can also help to treat cellulite too. I wouldn't waste any money on cellulite creams as I'm not convinced they work – cutting out caffeine and drinking more water is probably a more effective treatment for cellulite.

Baby soft skin

Apply a body oil straight after your shower, when your skin is still damp. The oil will seal in the moisture better.

Breakouts

When breakouts occur, I find **Bepanthen** nappy cream works a treat. Pop it on your spot after you've cleansed before bedtime.

Soft, supple lips

Give your lips a little exfoliation by using a specific lip scrub once a week. You can make your own scrub by mixing together brown sugar and olive oil. It works brilliantly. I like keeping a really soft toothbrush especially for giving my lips a little brush too.

Luscious lashes

If you're afraid of false lashes, don't be. They can really make the eyes look soft, big and beautiful. If you're a novice and a little nervous, go for the individual lashes. Do your eye make-up first and put on your mascara. Then, starting from the outside, pop on maybe three or four clusters, just on the outer corners. This is all you'll need to make a big difference.

 TIP *The glue that comes in the lash pack is usually useless. Get yourself some* **Duo** *lash adhesive glue, it's the best for sticking them.*

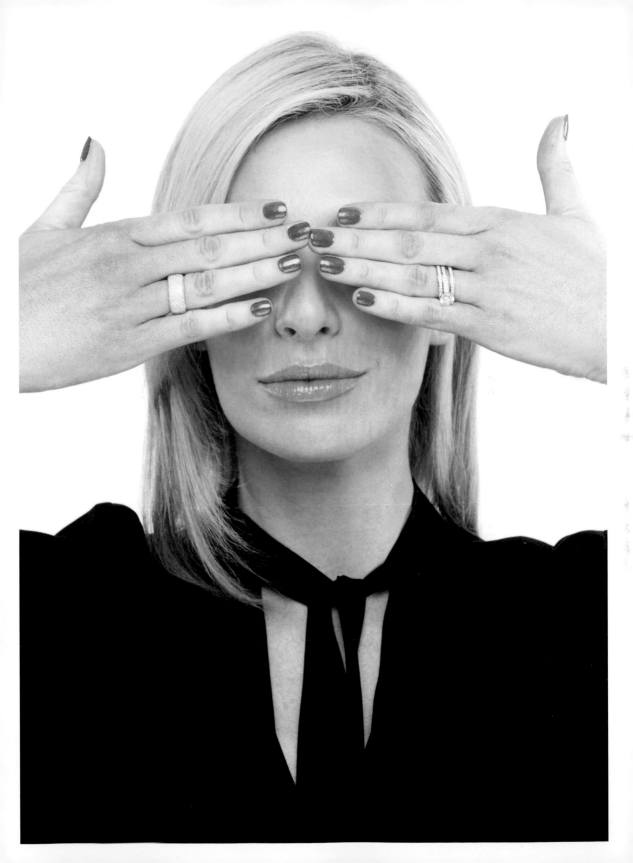

TANNING

I love having a glow to my skin but, being fair and freckly, this doesn't come easily to me. It also doesn't help that I live in Ireland, where, I think it's fair to say, sunbathing weather is pretty infrequent, even in the summer months!

Saying that, I'm not a great fan of lying in the sun. Even when I go on holiday I don't bother trying to get a real tan, partly because I'm so pale I'd need to be there for a month to get any kind of decent colour. Most importantly, it's because a real sun tan can be so bad for your skin.

Growing up, I was less worried about the effects of sun damage – which is often the way when you're young. Some of my girlfriends went on sunbeds like it was no big deal, and I did it once but never again as my mum went ballistic. And if somebody told me now they were going on a sunbed I'd think they were mad! Added to the fact that excessive exposure to the sun or the UV rays from a sunbed increases your risk of skin cancer, it can also be very ageing on your skin. There's nothing worse than leathery looking skin, particularly on someone's face.

All year round I wear an SPF on my face. I think this is key in protecting yourself from harmful rays but also it definitely helps with the ageing process. If you take two women in their fifties side by side – both with similar lifestyle habits but one wearing SPF all year round and one using it only in the summer months – I guarantee you'll notice a big difference in their skin's appearance.

On holidays or in the summer I always wear factor 50 on my face and at least a 30 on my body. So, my answer to achieving a golden tan? Fake it, baby!

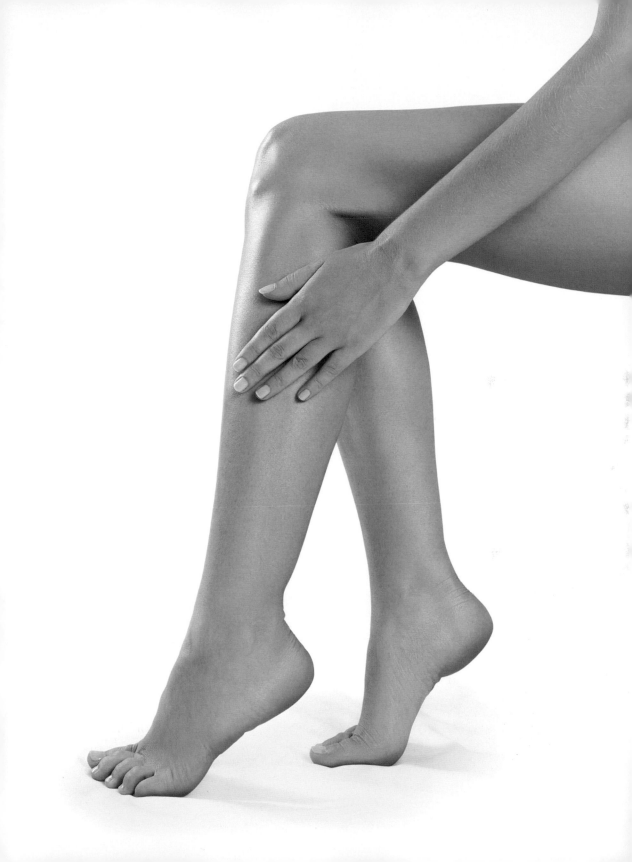

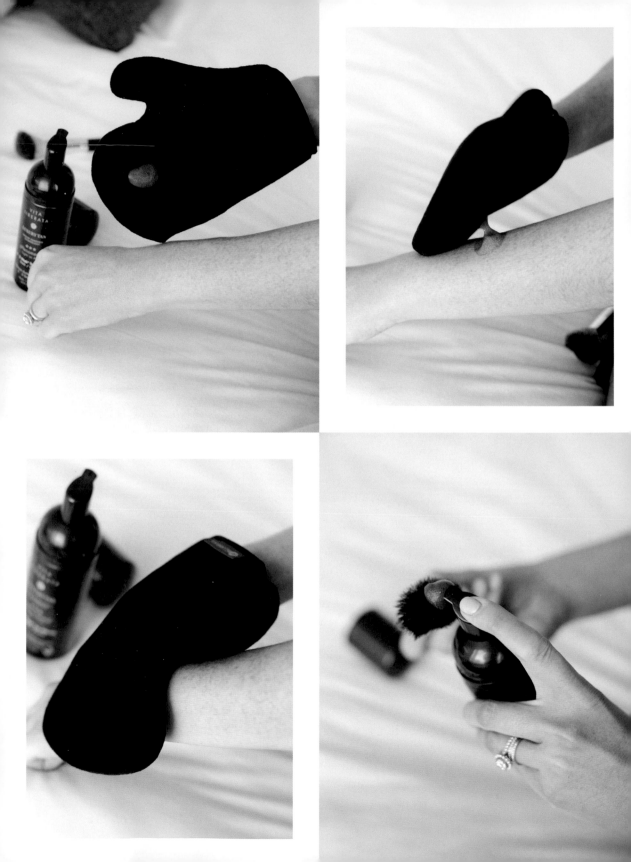

HOW TO ACHIEVE THAT PERFECT FAKE TAN

What you need:

My favourite type of tan is a dark tinted mouse as you can see what you're doing, it's quick to apply and quick to dry. I love **Vita Liberata pHenomenal 2–3 Week Self Tan**. It lasts really well on me and always fades gradually without any patches. A more budget-friendly one that is also very good is **Cocoa Brown 1 Hour Instant Tan**. Whichever you go for, though, make sure you have a clean mitt or glove – a velvet double-sided mitt is my preference.

1 First you need a good base, so exfoliating is key. You should exfoliate at least 12 hours before you apply your tan (I tend to exfoliate in the morning and then apply my tan in the evening). Exfoliate regularly to avoid build up, as several layers of tan can cause patchy skin. I like to use a good body scrub (**Cocoa Brown Tough Stuff** is great), along with an exfoliating mitt. I prefer a mitt to those cheap gloves as I find they're too harsh on my skin.

2 If you wax or shave, do it at least 24 hours before applying your tan.

3 Fake tan can be very drying and this causes it to go patchy, so it's important to give yourself a good layer of moisturizer the night before applying your tan. You can moisturize any problem areas like elbows, knees and feet immediately prior to tanning, too, if you feel you need it.

4 When you apply your tan, stand in front of a full-length mirror as you do it and take your time. If you rush it, you're bound to mess it up. When you do your face, mix some moisturizer in with your tan. Your face doesn't need to be as tanned as your body if you wear make-up.

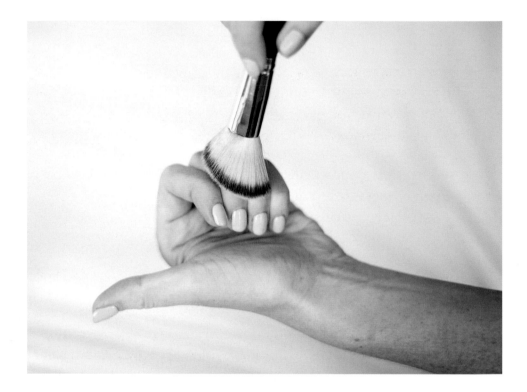

5 I always use an old foundation brush to tan my hands. Pump some tan onto your brush, hold your hand in a claw shape and lightly paint your hand and fingers. A little goes a long way here, so don't put too much product onto the brush. Blend in well between the fingers and at the sides of your palms.

6 When you've finished applying your tan, give yourself a few minutes before dressing. Wear loose clothing and avoid putting any tight underwear on.

7 To maintain the tan, apply some gradual tanning moisturizer every two to three days. On the other days, don't forget to use your normal body moisturizer as usual to help prevent the tan going patchy.

PAMPER NIGHT

Life can get hectic and stressful, so a nice pamper session every now and then is pretty necessary to keep ourselves sane! When you've had a busy working week and the weekend comes around, is there anything better than taking an hour or two out to pamper yourself?

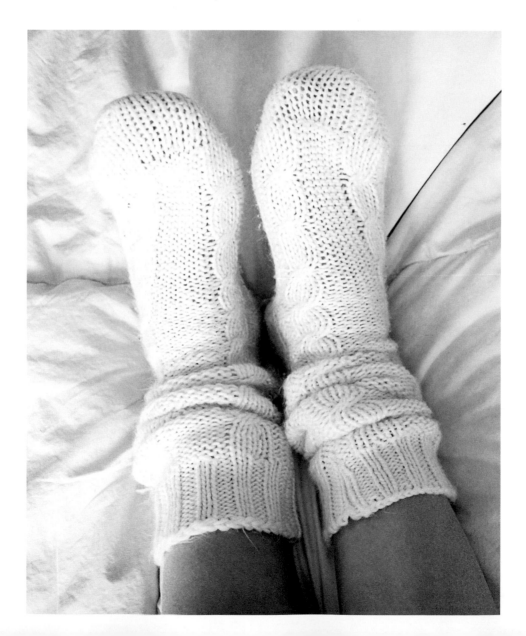

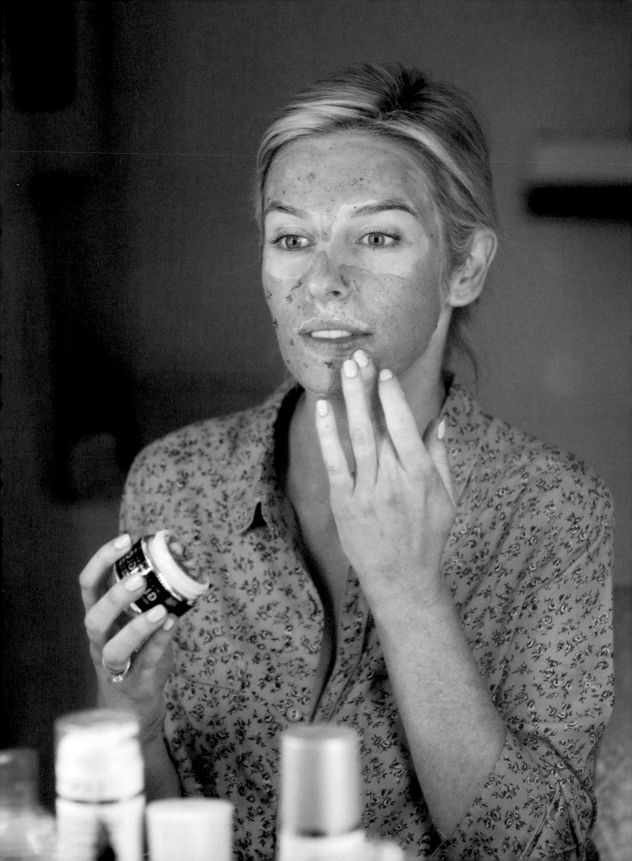

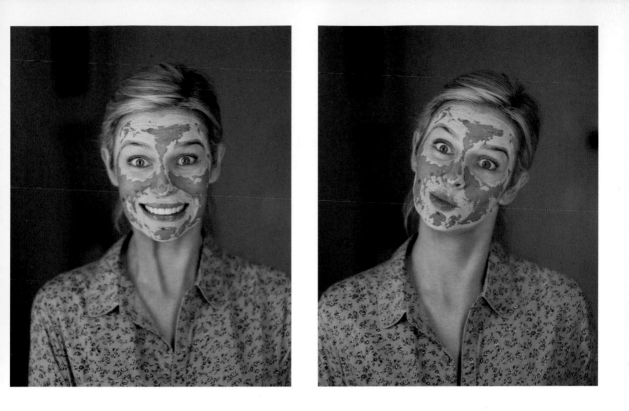

First things first, I light a candle (or three!). Then, while my bubble bath is running, I love to put on a face mask – my usual preference is **Glamglow Youthmud Tinglexfoliate Face Mask**. Leave it on your face for ten minutes, and when you wash it off your skin will feel sooo soft and fresh … I promise you. You can also apply a homemade face mask – these are really easy to create and great for the skin too (see recipes on page 133). Then, I like to apply the **Glamglow Thirstymud**, which really hydrates and calms the skin. It smells fab, too, fyi. Your face will be in tip-top condition!

It's always a good idea to exfoliate your body while you're in the bath just to get rid of dead skin cells or any leftover or unwanted tan. After the bath, I generously apply a body cream all over – I like **Kiehl's Creme de Corps** – it moisturizes the skin well and soaks in easily. No waiting around time before you get into your jammies!

For my hair, I like to apply a hair treatment – choose a mask of your choice (see pages 192–93) depending on what your hair needs. I wrap my hair in a hot towel and leave it for an hour or so. Or, when I'm feeling lazy, I tie my hair up and leave it in overnight. You can apply your mask to dry or damp hair.

I'll then apply my usual eye cream followed by an oil for my face – I love using oils at nighttime. **Clarins Blue Orchid Face Treatment** oil is a good one. After that, it's time for lip balm. **Nuxe Reve de Miel** is one of my all time faves. You can use this every day (I usually do) but it's lovely to apply before bed, too!

What pamper night would be complete without snuggling up in cosy PJs and fluffy socks? Sometimes I'll apply an extra layer of moisturizer to my feet before I put on my fluffy socks – this really makes them soft by morning.

And then last but not least, I pour myself a nice glass of wine and munch on some chocolate … Ah, bliss!

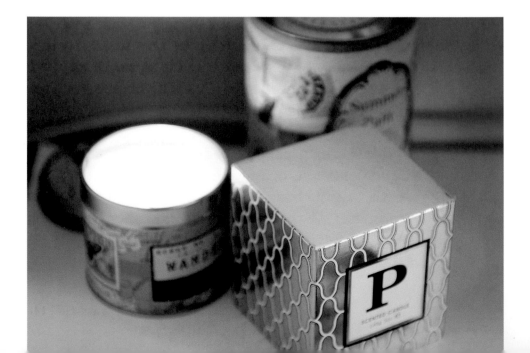

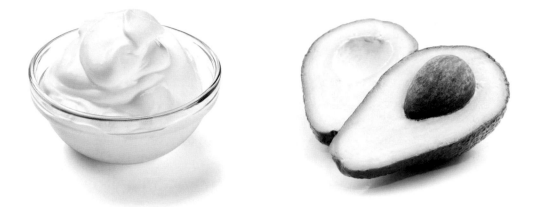

FACE MASKS

Here are a few face masks you can make up at home, all of which will nourish and brighten your skin.

Avocado & yoghurt

Mash ¼ ripe **avocado**. Mix in ½ teaspoon of **honey** and 1 teaspoon of plain organic **yoghurt** to make a paste. Apply to face and leave it on for 10-15 minutes. Rinse with lukewarm water.

Banana

Mash ½ **banana**. Mix in a tablespoon of **orange juice** and a tablespoon of **honey**. Apply to the face and leave it on for 10–15 minutes. Rinse with lukewarm water.

Oatmeal

Mix ¼ cup hot (not boiling) water and ⅓ cup **oatmeal**. Mix in 2 tablespoons of plain **yoghurt**, 2 tablespoons of **honey** and 1 small **egg white**. Apply the mixture to the face and let it sit for 10–15 minutes. Rinse with lukewarm water.

HOW TO FAKE SLIMMER LEGS WITH A BEAUTIFUL SHIMMER

I love tanned legs but I also love that it's possible to enhance the length and shape of your legs too. Yes! And it doesn't involve a diet.

My skin is very fair – or you could say ghostly white with lots of freckles! (Although I do love the freckles.) So, in the summer or if I'm going anywhere with bare legs, I always like to give them a bit of colour. I love using mousse to tan as it's quick, easy and you can see where you're applying it as it's tinted.

So, before I go to bed, I use a light layer of dark mousse on my legs. I apply a good layer of the mousse with a clean tanning mitt and leave to develop overnight. The next morning, I gently shower it all off.

TIP *If you shave your legs, don't apply your tan straightaway – shave them in the morning and then apply the tan in the evening.*

Then, I apply a layer of **E45 Intense Recovery moisturizer**. This is for very dry skin but I think it's a brilliant everyday moisturizer and suitable for most skin types. It's especially good if you're often applying tan, as this can be drying on the legs. I sometimes get red dots on my legs after putting instant tan on, and the E45 helps to prevent this by adding a barrier effect to the skin, leaving the legs very shiny and smooth looking. It's the perfect base for what's to follow …

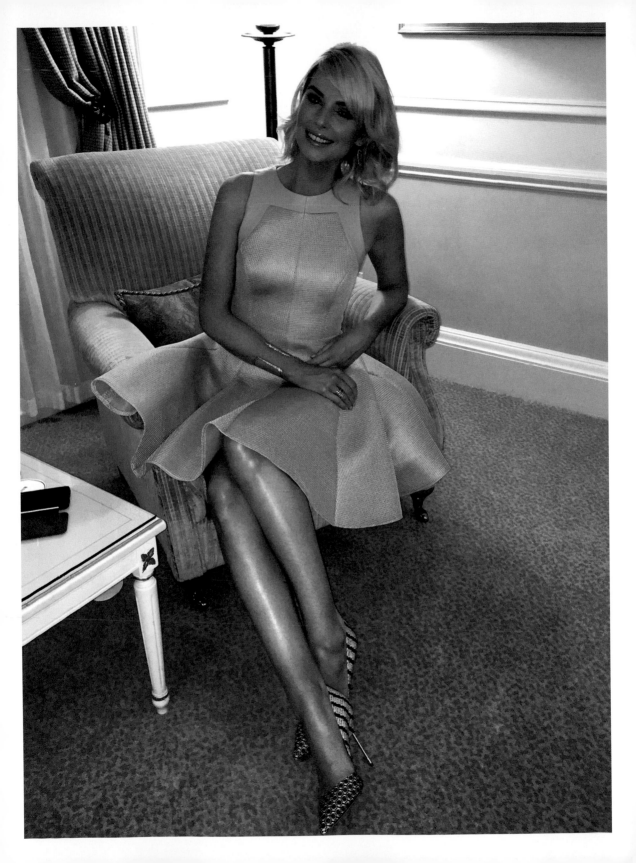

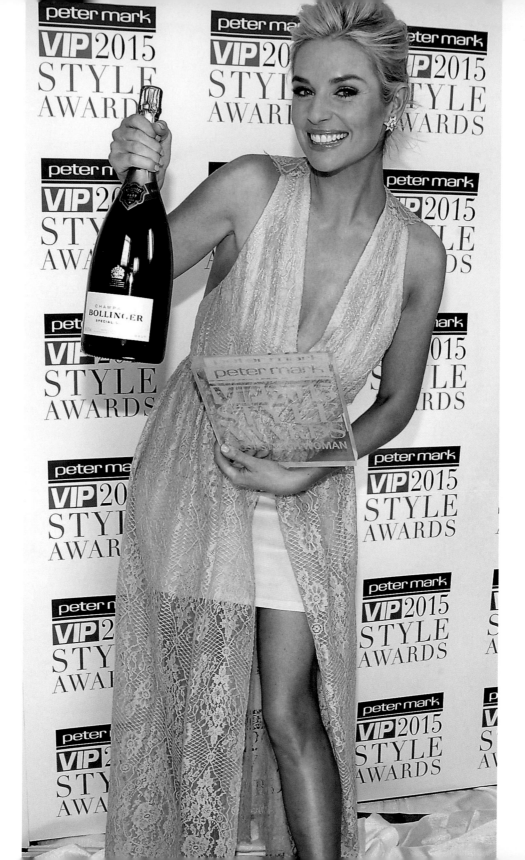

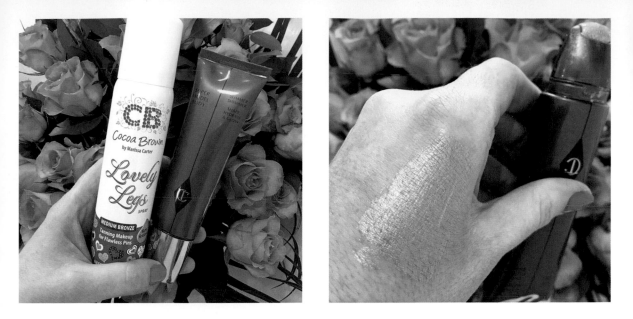

At night, before I get dressed to go out, I spray a light layer of **Cocoa Brown Lovely Legs** (on top of the mousse I've put on the night before). It's an instant tan, like make-up for the legs. I rub that in using the mitt from before. Then, last but not least, it's my ultimate leg product: **Charlotte Tilbury Supermodel Body Slimmer Shimmer**.

This is my absolute favourite product for achieving glistening skin. It really gives your legs the most fabulous sheen. I apply it down the centre of my legs – its rolling applicator makes it easy to apply. I actually buff it in with a clean foundation brush. Yes, I literally paint myself!

It makes legs appear longer and slimmer – honestly it does, and I've seen the result on other people too. I also use it on my arms, back and collarbones. It's stunning on the skin and I think it would be beautiful on brides, too, especially if they're wearing a strapless dress. I used something similar on my wedding day.

There are other products you can use, too, like **Victoria's Secret Rockin' Body Leg Shine**, and the Body Shop also has a lovely coconut body butter with a shimmer.

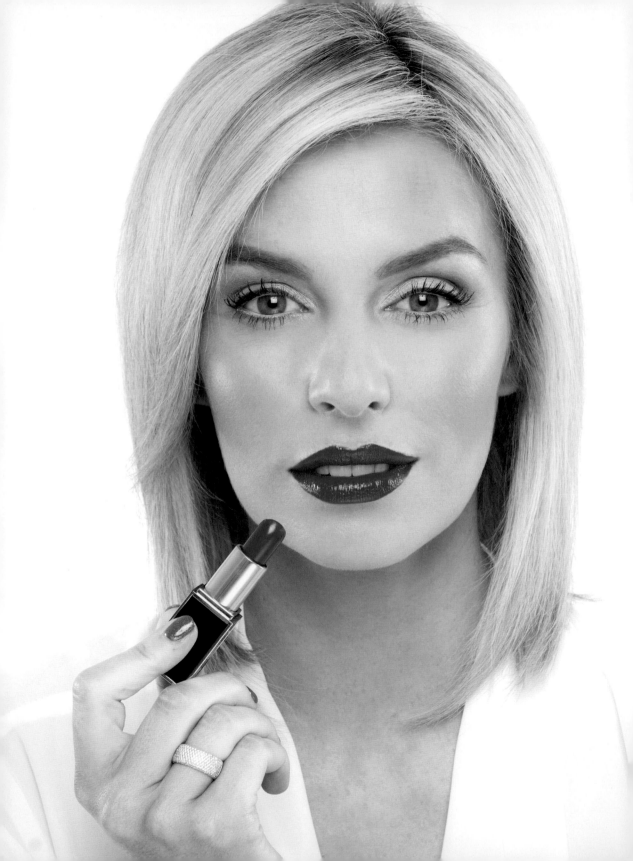

CHAPTER FIVE

MAKE-UP

I adore make-up. I love how you can create such different looks to suit your mood or occasion. It can emphasize your best features and give you a youthful glow in seconds and there are so many fantastic products out there. I like a fresh, natural look during the day but it's great to go for something with a little more impact when I'm out in the evening or at a special event. Over the years I've picked up lots of tips from make-up professionals, and some of the best ones are included in this chapter.

At home, it's important to have the right equipment and kit – a good selection of make-up brushes is an absolute must! Choose products that suit your skin type and colouring – and they don't necessarily need to blow your budget. Knowing just a few simple techniques can also make a huge difference, from easy eyeliner tricks to how to apply your make-up in just ten minutes. Even contouring your face for a defined, sculpted look might seem like one for the experts but it is in fact easy to achieve. Give it a go and have some fun with your make-up!

FOUNDATION

Foundation has to be one of a woman's best friends. A beautiful base is everything to me. I love beautifully flawless and glowing skin. I really dislike heavy, caked, matte-looking skin. I just think it's ageing on everyone. People shouldn't be afraid of foundation but equally shouldn't feel the need to trowel it on. Your skin should still be visible through foundation, and if, like me, you have freckles, embrace them and don't try to hide them.

Growing up, I used pan sticks that were heavy, greasy and orange in colour. Everything about it was wrong. There's nothing worse than seeing pretty young girls with faces covered in orange foundation. A perfect foundation should make your skin look its best by perfecting uneven skin tone, making it appear bright, clear and youthful.

There are lots of formulas to choose from so, again, it's down to preference and deciding what you want from your foundation. Again, it's important to know your skin type. If you've got oily skin, it's best to go for a foundation that is oil-free. If you have dry skin, you'll want something labelled hydrating or dewy, and if you've normal to combination skin, you have a little more choice. If you do have dry skin, make sure it's well-moisturized and primed before you apply your foundation.

In the summer, I like tinted moisturizers as they're light and easy to use. They can be applied with your fingers with no fuss and are ideal for anyone who doesn't want anything too heavy on their skin.

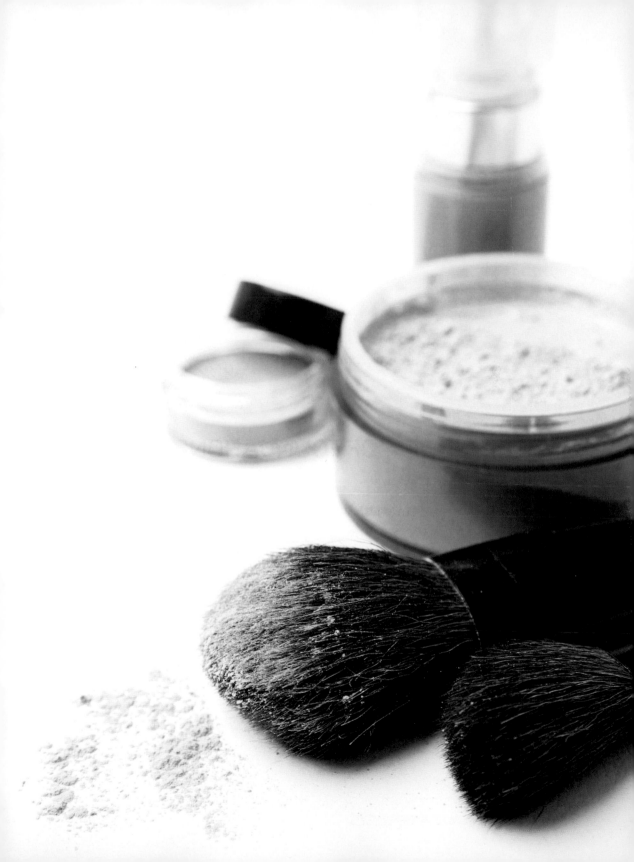

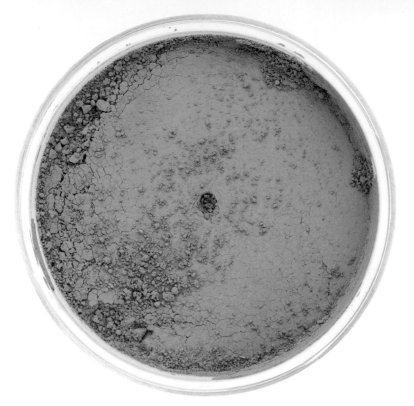

TYPES OF FOUNDATIONS

Mineral foundations

I would usually recommend mineral make-up (I like **Bare Minerals**) to women with very sensitive or acne-prone skin. Made from tiny particles of minerals, this kind of make-up is free from chemicals and additives, so it's less likely to cause any skin irritation. Mineral make-up is also good for teenagers, and the mineral powder is easy to apply.

Powder foundations

Powders 'set' your foundation, helping it last longer. I like powder foundations for touch ups while I'm out. I wouldn't solely use a powder foundation personally as I don't feel I get a flawless overall finish. They come in a compact, making them ideal for your handbag. I really like **Mac Studio Fix** for when I'm on the go.

Liquid foundations

A liquid foundation is the most common one women choose. It's my number one choice too. I like my liquid foundation to be medium in coverage and not heavy-looking. I like a dewy, luminescent feel. One of my favourites is **Armani Luminous Silk**. This photographs beautifully too. A cheaper but excellent alternative to the Armani is **L'Oreal True Match**, although I wouldn't recommend that one to someone with dry skin. A gorgeous oil-free option is **Stila Stay All Day**.

I always apply my foundation with a buffing brush. That's just my preference – I find a flat brush can leave streaks. I rarely use my fingers, unless I'm in a hurry or in the mood to get them dirty!

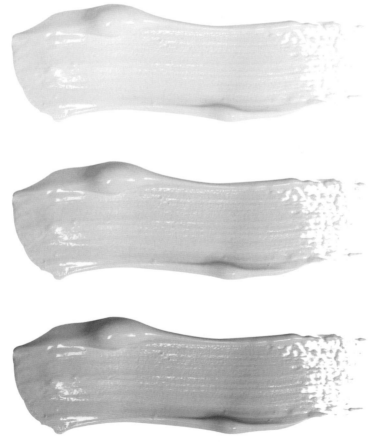

HOW TO APPLY YOUR FOUNDATION

Apply your foundation bit by bit – you often need much less than you think. I work from the nose and cheek area outwards. Make sure you blend well around the jawline, keeping everything soft – you don't want harsh lines anywhere – and be careful around your nose. I tend not to apply foundation right under the eyes, as I prefer to leave this area free for concealer. Apply your foundation in good light, so you can ensure everything blends in properly. We probably all look better by candlelight, but our make-up coverage needs to work in bright lights and the daytime too!

What shade to go for

I find a yellow-based foundation suits nearly everybody unless you're extremely pale, in which case you're probably in the cool pink category. Generally, though, I just don't find pinks as flattering as the yellow-based shades.

If you're buying from a pharmacy or shop and you have no assistance I suggest you pick out the three shades that you think will work on you. Never sample a shade on your hand to get your correct shade. Your hand is a different colour to your face.

Apply a small amount of each onto your jawline using your finger. You should then go for the colour that disappears. Don't go for the the colour you want to be! Often we opt for darker shades because we want to look darker but, trust me, don't do that. You can always warm up your skin colour with bronzer afterwards. Apply a little more of the foundation colour you're happy with – go to the light or preferably outside to look in a mirror. Lights in stores can be deceiving.

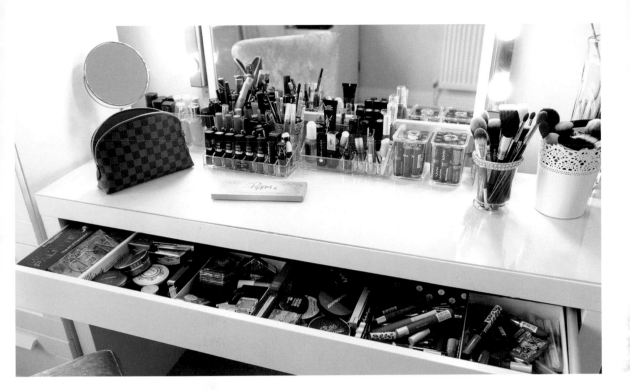

If you can, I think it's best to go to a beauty counter and ask the sales assistants for help. Wear little or no make-up, and ask for two or three shades to be tested on your skin. Again, look at them in natural light. Foundation takes at least thirty minutes to settle into the skin, so you could go for a coffee and then take another look at how it sits and feels before buying anything. Never feel pressured to purchase there and then. Also, ask for samples – all the counters have them. If you're spending good money on a foundation you have to be sure you're happy with it, so don't be shy.

TIP *If you're a tanning lover, it's best to invest in two foundation shades. One for everyday wear and one a little darker for your nights out when you're wearing fake tan.*

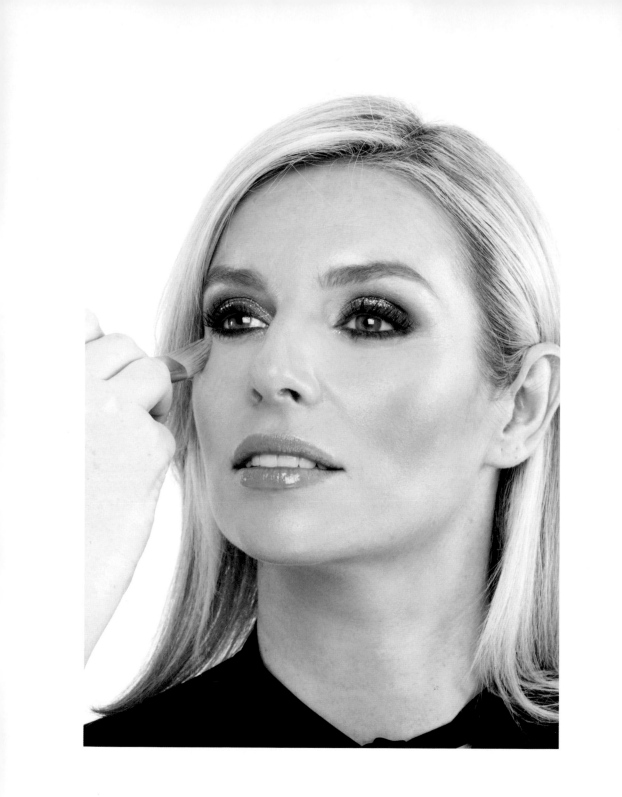

CONCEALERS

Concealers are a girl's best friend and really help to hide blemishes, reduce dark circles and brighten under the eyes generally. Always use them after you have applied your foundation. I opt for a liquid concealer in a tube, applying it with the applicator or my fingers, and buffing it smooth with a little concealer brush. I have concealers in varying shades for different areas I'm trying to cover up:

Spots & redness

You need a concealer the same shade as your foundation, as a lighter shade will only highlight the area more. **Stila Stay All Day Foundation**, which I already mentioned, is great as it has a concealer to match the foundation in the lid.

Dark circles under the eyes

To counteract the blue/grey colour under the eyes you should opt for a light to medium peach colour if you're fair skinned. If you have dark skin go for a dark or orange colour.

Brighten and highlight

To brighten under the eyes and give yourself a facelift in seconds (as my make-up artist friend Tara always says) try this simple step – use a lightweight concealer in a shade lighter than your foundation. I like **Urban Decay Naked Skin Concealer** for this. Draw an upside-down triangle shape under the eye, with the tip of the triangle pointing downwards. Get your concealer brush (I like a fluffy small-headed one for this) and blend everything up and outwards. This will instantly lift and brighten the area.

PRIMERS

Primers, which are applied after you've moisturized but before your foundation, create a soft layer and smooth out your skin texture. They've become pretty popular in the last couple of years, but not everyone needs them, in my opinion. Saying that, if you suffer from oily skin and large open pores, or if you find your make-up slides off your face during the day, then primers could be an essential item in your make-up kit. Primers can also colour correct skin, reducing redness, and my favourite one is **Stila One Step Corrector**.

 TIP *For a quick fix, you can mix your primer in with your moisturizer – a small pea-sized amount is all you need. Apply in one go, before doing your make-up.*

Eyeshadow primer is another product that's not essential but definitely worth having, in my opinion. An eyeshadow primer goes on before you apply anything to your eyelids, and only a tiny amount is needed. A good eyeshadow primer should prevent shadows from falling into your creases. Our eyelids are naturally quite oily so, if you find your shadow is creasing a lot, a primer is for you. It can also help to bring out the intensity of the colour you're applying. My favourite eyeshadow primer is **Urban Decay Primer Potion**.

 TIP *If you haven't got any eyeshadow primer, try patting a small amount of concealer onto the lids, then set it with translucent powder – this can do the trick too.*

SETTING POWDER

A good setting powder is a must in my opinion, especially if you find your base is not lasting or is going patchy throughout the day. I like to use a translucent setting powder. **Laura Mercier** does a fabulous one and it really works well. You should look for something colourless and very fine in texture.

You only need to lightly pat your powder onto your T-zone – be very light-handed with this step. You can then invest in a cheaper translucent powder in a compact form for your bag.

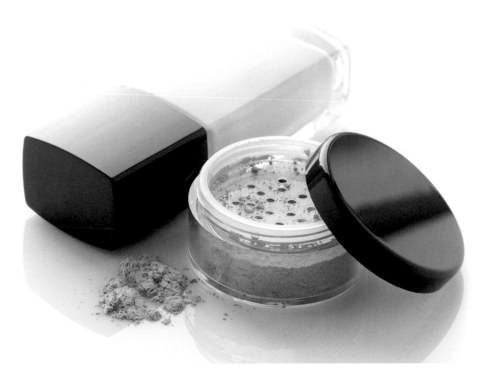

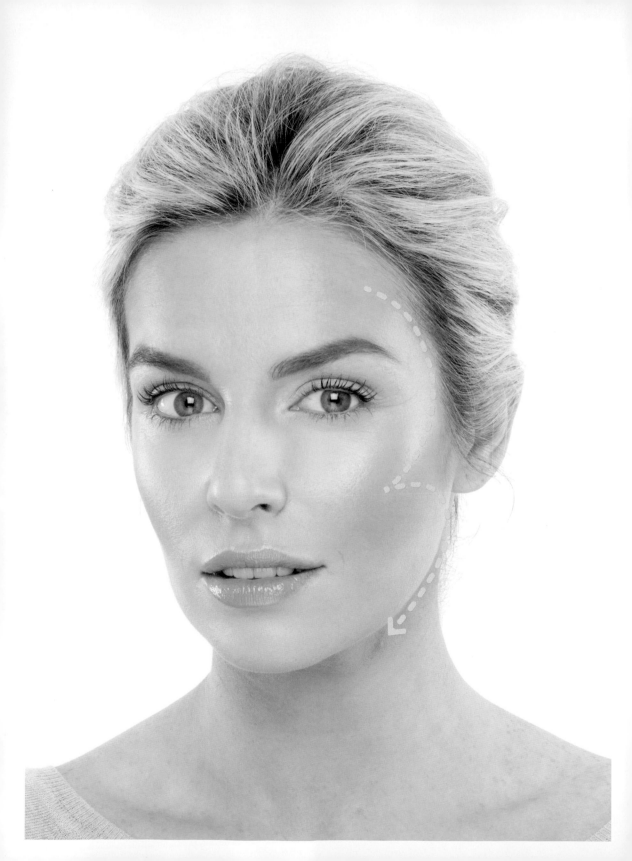

CONTOURING

Contouring can help to sculpt and define the face. It's a fantastic look but I hate that it's been made to seem scary and only for the advanced. (This is probably down to the Kardashians showing their faces painted with creamy stripes.)

Contouring with creams is definitely trickier than using powders, and if done incorrectly can make you look like you've smeared brown muck on your face. I personally don't use creams to contour. I think they work really well for a photoshoot, or for a special event, but for everyday use a powder is more practical and can take seconds to apply.

Here's how I contour:

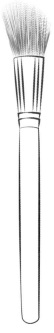

1 First, I dust my favourite shimmer-free bronzer onto my brush (see my brush images on pages 166–67). You should only use a matte shade to contour. I use Amour from my own palette every day as it's the perfect cool brown shade.

2 Starting from the hollow part under my cheekbone I lightly brush out to my hairline. Then, moving to my temples, I simply sweep the colour in the figure of a three on each side of my face. So, from temples to under your cheekbone to under your jawline.

3 Repeat the step depending on how chiselled and Gisele-like you want to be!!

TOP 10 MAKE-UP PRODUCTS
EVERYONE NEEDS

1 **BB cream or an illuminating balm**
Both products (BB stands for beauty balm, or blemish balm) can brighten your complexion to give your skin a healthy glow.

2 **Concealer**
For those blemishes or dark eye circles.

3 **Mascara**
Enhances your eyes with darker, more defined eyelashes.

4 **Nude eyeliner**
Takes away any redness from the waterline (the lower lash line), and makes eyes appear bigger, rounder and brighter.

5 **Matte eyeshadow**
A staple eyeshadow for all make-up kits.

6 **Matte bronzer**
Contours your face in a matter of seconds.

7 **Nude lipstick**
There are dozens of different shades – something for everyone.

8 **Blusher**
Gives you a bit of colour and youthfulness.

9 **Golden powder highlighter**
I love highlighter and couldn't do without this. Putting it on the brow bone and into the tear duct makes all the difference.

10 **Eyebrow pencil**
Defines and enhances your brows. I like soft, waxy pencils. Charlotte Tilbury's **Shape, Lift and Shade Tool** or Mac's **Brow Definer** are excellent.

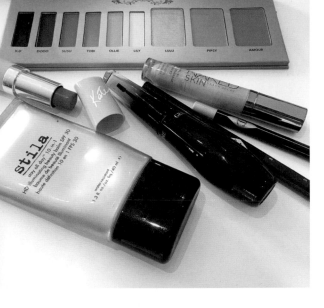
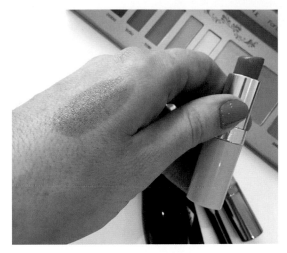
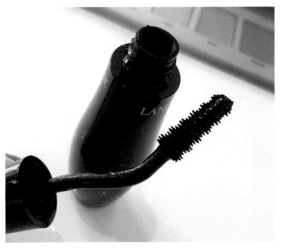
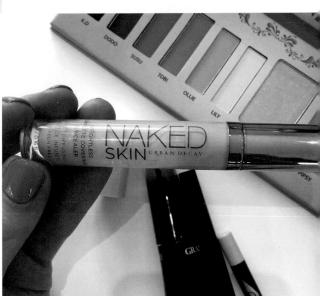
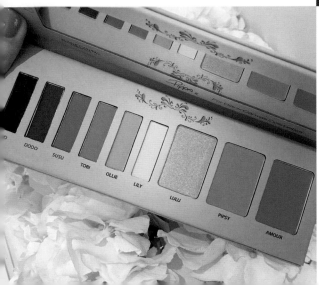
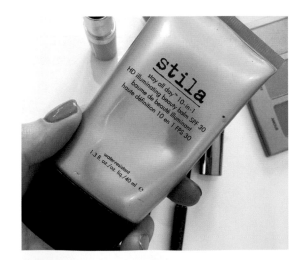

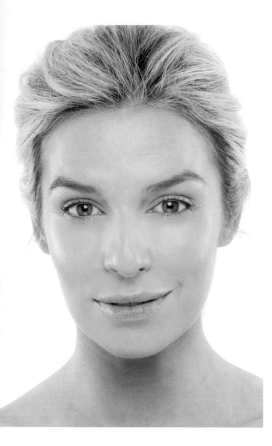

HOW TO DO YOUR MAKE-UP IN TEN MINUTES

If, like me, you only have ten minutes to get ready most mornings, this simple guide should help you get out the door. I think the key to getting your make-up done quickly in the morning is to be organized. If my make-up table is in a mess and I can't see what I need, it slows me down, and puts me in a bad mood!

So organize your make-up the night before and make sure your brushes are clean and close to hand. The make-up that you use every day should be in one place and easy to see. Once that's done, you're ready to go – here's how I do it:

- I mix together moisturizer and primer in my hand, then dab a small amount onto my skin and buff it in. *(30 seconds)*

- If it's summer, I'll use my illuminating balm or BB cream – in the winter, or if I want more coverage, I'll use my liquid foundation. I always use a brush to apply it, but you could do this with your fingers – just make sure they're clean. *(2 mins)*

- Then it's concealer if I'm covering any spots. I'll always highlight under my eyes with a lighter concealer. *(1 min)*

- A quick sweep of setting powder. *(30 seconds)*

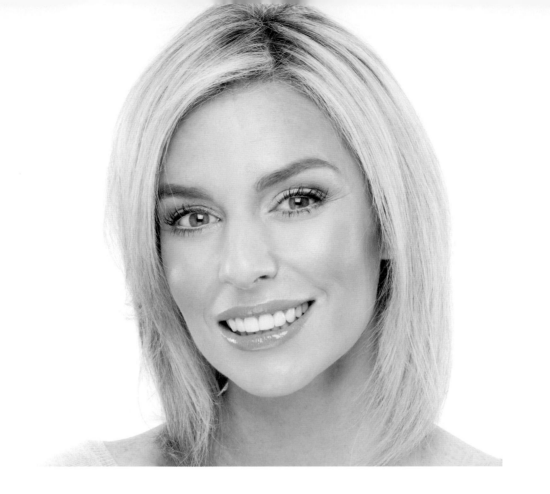

- Then I'll contour my face in a figure of three. *(2 min)*

- I'll then fill in my brows using an eyebrow pencil or 'Susu' from the Pippa Palette. *(1 min)*

- Next it's my eyes. For eyeshadow, I use **Tobi** (a warm matte brown) or **Lili** (a soft creamy colour) from the Pippa Palette. Just one shade all over each lid and buffed into the crease. *(1 min)*

- Nude liner on my waterline to open the eyes. *(30 seconds)*

- A quick lick of mascara. *(30 seconds)*

- A pop of blusher. *(30 seconds)*

- Gloss or nude lippy. *(30 seconds)*   **Done!**

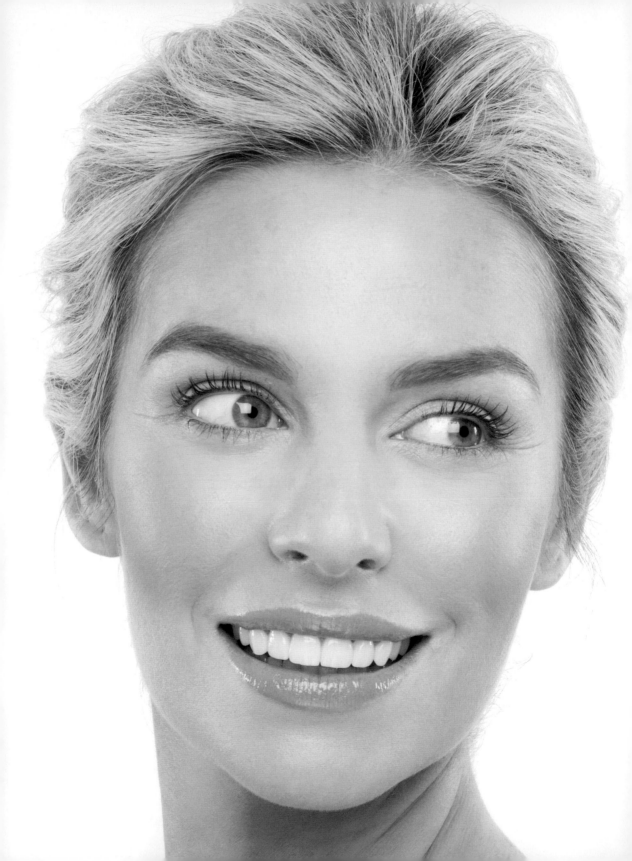

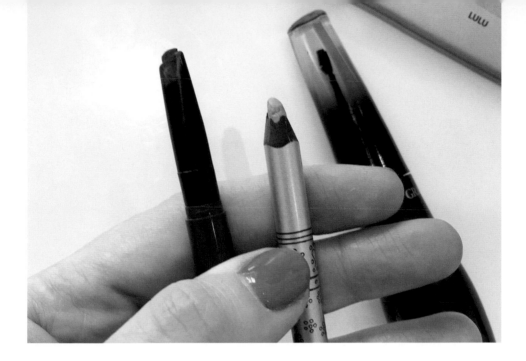

HOW TO ACHIEVE BIG BRIGHT EYES

I've learned lots of tips and tricks over the years about how to look fresher and brighter just with a few beauty products. This morning, for example, my alarm woke me at 5.30 a.m. My eyes were in the back of my head and I felt like I'd only been asleep for an hour at most. I hate that feeling!

So, here are a few little cheats that I love and swear by, to make your eyes look big and bright. They're really quick to do, too – bonus!

1 Nude eyeliner

I cannot stress how important nude liner is for every woman. You absolutely must buy one if you don't own one. Our waterline (the lower lash line) is red naturally, but when we're tired it looks even redder. A nude liner will instantly make your eyes look fresher and bigger. I rarely wear a black liner in my waterline – nine times out of ten, I opt for nude – even when I want a smoky eye.

My two favourites are:

- **Charlotte Tilbury Eye Cheat** – it's the most expensive nude liner I've used but it's the best. It doesn't budge so you won't have to reapply.
- A close second favourite is the **Stila Kajal** liner.

2 Mascara

My first rule here is replace your mascara every three months. Beyond that time they'll just dry up and you'll have clumpy-looking lashes. Plus they're unhygienic after three months. So, bin yours and purchase a fresh one if it's had its day.

I don't believe in spending money on mascaras especially since you only get a few months out of one, so just go for any of the affordable pharmacy brands. **Rimmel** or **L'Oreal** would be my brands of choice for mascara.

3 Brow lifter

So, on make-up days, I use my mascara, nude liner and usually this little product. A brow lifter, which usually looks like a big pencil with a creamy, pearlized colour on one end, will define brow arches and highlight them. I like to use **Anastasia Beverly Hills Brow Duality**, which is a highlighting pencil that I use on the brow bone. It lifts the brow while subtly highlighting too. This one contains a matte crayon or a shimmer crayon.

4 A golden highlighter

A highlighter (like **Lulu** from my palette) popped onto your tear duct will instantly open up your eyes.

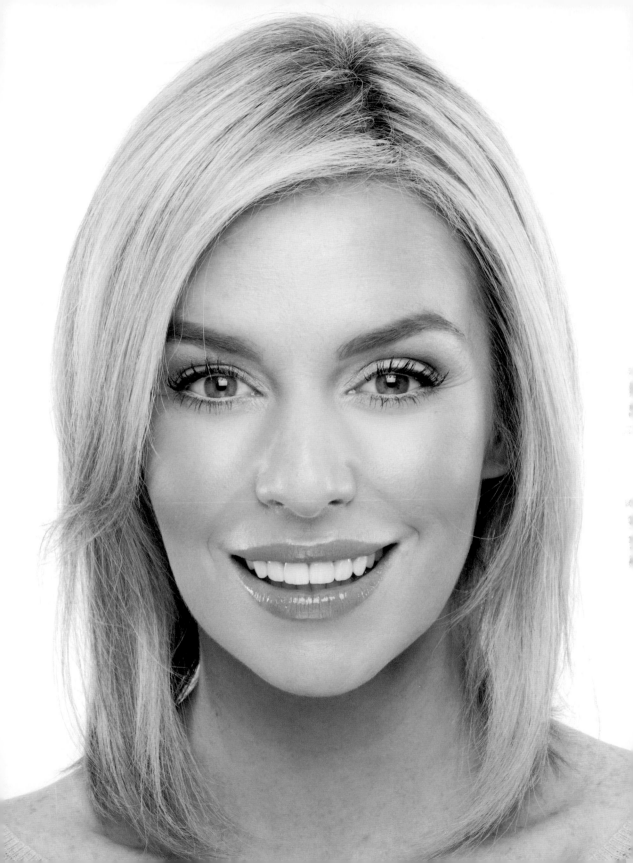

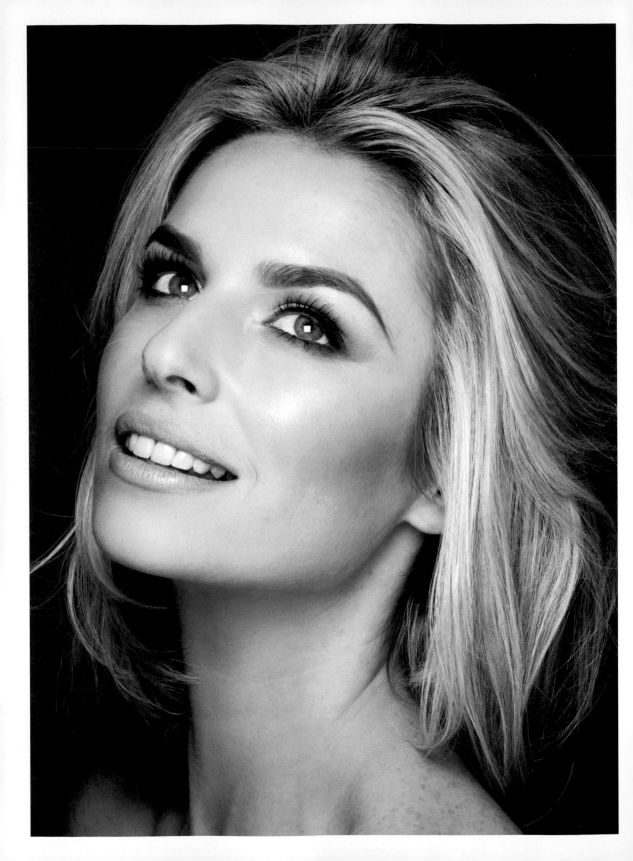

BROWS

Ladies! Let's talk brows and their importance. Take it from me, they can change the look of your entire face. Just look at how mine used to be.

I know this picture of me years ago is so embarrassing but, hey, it's online anyway so I may as well show it here too and we can all laugh together. (Cringe!)

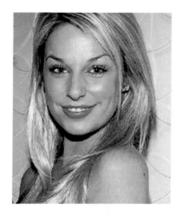

I, like many other people, totally over plucked my brows. They were way too arched as well, which I didn't need to emphasize, as they're naturally quite high and arched anyhow. Over-arching them made it look like I was constantly surprised.

So, how did I get them thick and into a shape that suits my face? First, I went to an HD Pro Brow artist. The HD brow method involves tinting, waxing and threading – it's a precision procedure that transforms your brows into the perfect shape for your face, enhancing your facial features. It's not just shaping and tidying. It sculpts your brows into the perfect shape, whether they are overgrown or over-plucked.

Eyebrow Embroidery is another option. This procedure lasts between 12 and 18 months. This creates a really natural look, thickening or darkening existing eyebrows and making them more defined by strategically placing 3D hair strokes on the top layer of the skin. It's therefore more superficial than tattooing.

I go to HD brow artist Kim O'Sullivan who is based in the Dublin Make-up Academy. Kim is a brow genius and I've seen her work wonders on many people (me included).

And now my brows are in a shape I'm happy with, I only have to visit Kim every few months and maintain them myself in between. Here's what I use on my brows:

Gels

Brow gels help to define and neaten your brows. I love **Anastasia DipBrow** – I got mine in Sephora in America but you can get it online as well. The **Laura Mercier Brow Gel** is lovely too. My must-have brow brush to apply any brow gel is the **Blank Canvas E44**.

Shadow

An eyeshadow is a simple way to define your brows and the result is very natural. I often use **Susu** from my palette to fill mine in as it's a soft taupe-like colour. All you need is a thin flat eyebrush and to make sure you go for a shade that suits your natural colouring.

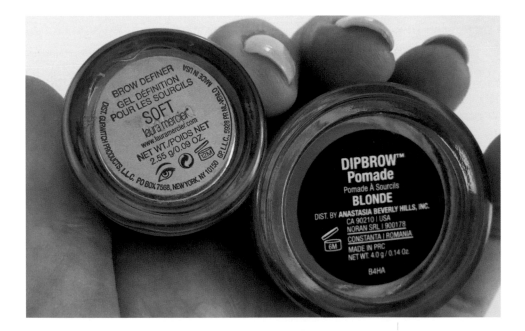

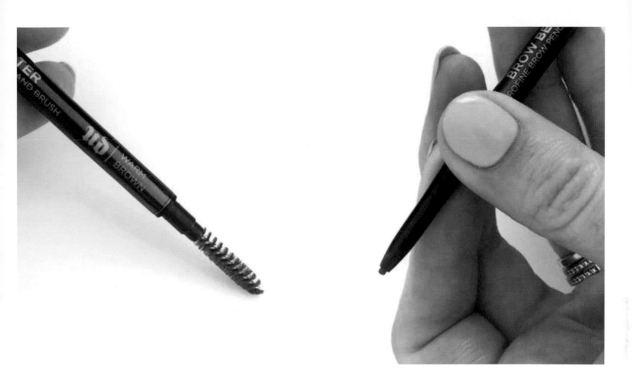

Pencil

You can also use a pencil to fill in your brows. **Urban Decay** have a product called **Brow Beater**. On one end you have a soft pencil that very easily glides onto the skin allowing you to achieve a really defined line. On the other end, you have a really handy brush. I always brush out my brows to soften them after I've used any product.

Brow setters

If you want to keep your brows in place while adding a tint of colour you'll love these. **Urban Decay Brow Tamer** or **Benefit's Gimme Brow** are my top two. These are like mascara for the brows. I really like them on their own, too, if you just want to quickly groom them and run. Which is me most days!

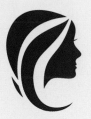

EXPERT TIPS: BROWS

Here also are some top tips from my very own HD brow expert, Kim O'Sullivan:

Take care when you tweeze!

When using tweezers, proceed with caution. Always tweeze two to three hairs up close then step away to look at your handiwork.

Don't get 'tweezer-happy', only to discover you've created a gap, or one brow is much thinner than the other. Never tweeze when you're angry or just looking for something to do – never take your emotions out on your eyebrows!

Find a highly-trained brow artist whom you can trust

Just like your hairdresser, it's so important that you build a rapport with your brow artist. They will get to know your brows' behaviour, that is their regrowth pattern. So many people make the mistake of going to a different brow artist on each visit. Always request the same artist.

Master the art of 'less is more'

Don't be heavy-handed. Using short featherlike strokes to mimic hairs, softly fill in any spaces and always comb through to blend out colour and soften harsh lines. Never overload your brush with product.

A good brow artist should explain how your brows are progressing and which parts need filling in. With a good angled brow brush, and your preferred brow product, filling them in should only take a few moments.

When defining your brows, concentrate the pigment intensity in the arch of your brow. This will create the illusion of a more lifted and youthful look. Finish off with a brow bone brightener under the entire brow, again focusing on the arch, and blend out with your pinky finger.

Set your brows to keep them in place

If you run out of your brow setting gel, spray a little hairspray onto your brow brush and comb through your brows. Not a hair will budge, I promise.

Get more staying power out your brow tint

To get more out of your tint in between visits, apply a thin layer of Vaseline to your brows before getting into the bath or shower to protect them and prevent the steam from leaching the tint out.

ESSENTIAL MAKE-UP BRUSHES

To apply make-up really well, you need a good selection of brushes. There are so many different types of brushes, varying in size and bristle type, each one helping you to achieve that perfect look. I tend to use natural-haired brushes for powders (so, for contouring, highlighting, blending and for eyeshadows) and brushes with synthetic hairs for liquids (so, for concealers or foundation). Here are the types of brushes that I think are essential for any make-up kit.

- **1) Foundation brush** – there's lots of choice here as they come in various sizes and shapes. My favourite is a flat buffing brush.

- **2) Contour/bronzer brush** – I use a small headed fluffy angled brush for contouring or bronzing.

- **3) Eyeshadow brush x 3** – you really only need three: a flat brush to place your product on the eyelid, a fluffy blending brush (very important) and a tiny pointy one for applying shadow on your bottom lash line or smudging your liner on your upper lash line.

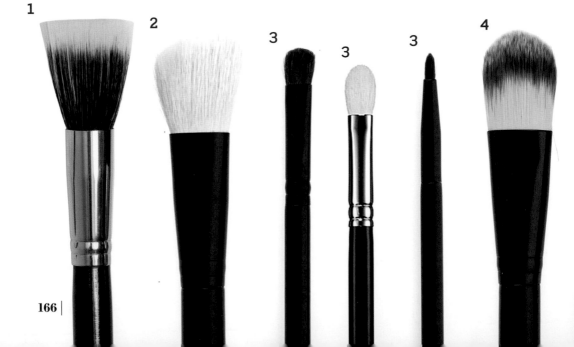

1   2   3   3   3   4

- **4) Highlighter brush** – you can use the same brush for contouring and highlighting if you don't want to double up. I use a smaller-headed fluffy brush with a slight point on the top.

- **5) Blusher brush** – use a small-headed fluffy brush for applying your blusher.

- **6) Brow brush** – a small, flat-angled brush is essential for filling in your brows with a shadow.

- **7) Powder brush** – to set your foundation you'll need a large fluffy brush. I like it to be pointed as well.

- **8) Concealer brush** – I like to use a small flat brush for concealing blemishes.

- **9) Lipbrush** (optional) – a small brush with a tip is good for applying strong, defined colour, especially red lipstick, on your lips.

- **10) Angled eyeliner brush** (optional) – if you're going to try any fancy flicks on your eyes, a slim, fine-tipped eyeliner brush is a must!

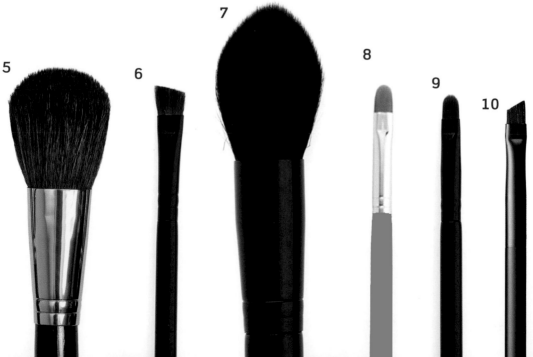

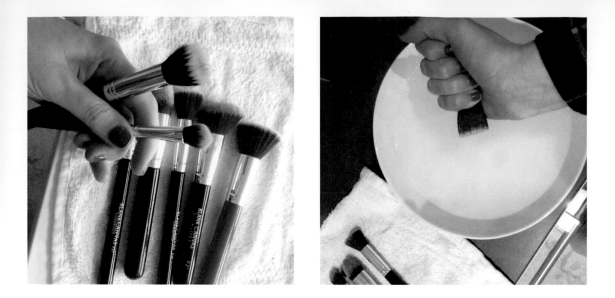

HOW TO WASH
YOUR MAKE-UP BRUSHES

When it comes to cleaning your make-up brushes, do you know how to clean them properly? Or, do you ever clean them? Go on – hands up who doesn't at all! Not many I'm guessing, so I thought I'd share a few tips on how to clean your brushes correctly.

First, it's really important to get into the routine of cleaning your brushes. Think about all the oil and dirt that accumulates on them, which you then brush onto your skin. A build-up of bacteria will lead to blocked pores and breakouts, so keeping your brushes clean is a definite must. Your brushes will also last longer if you look after them.

So, how often should you wash them? For me, it's once a week. Pick an evening every week and try to stick to it. If you have acne, I recommend washing them more often, maybe three times a week. You can also get a professional brush spray and use it daily in between your deep cleans. This will help to eliminate any bacteria gathering in your brushes. **Elf Daily Brush Cleaner** is good.

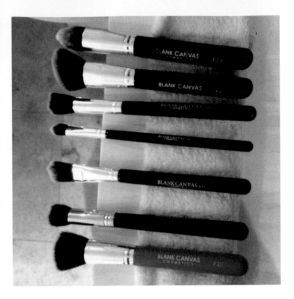

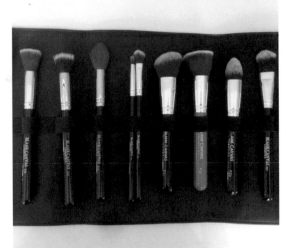

1. Fill a large bowl with tepid (not boiling) water and pour in a small amount of mild baby shampoo. I use one of Ollie's fragrance-free ones, like **Burt's Bees** or **Elave**.

2. Swirl the brush around the bowl – you'll immediately see the make-up come off – and rub the brush in the palm of your other hand until no more make-up is coming out of it. It's important to hold the ferrule (the metal part) and ensure you don't get that part wet. That's where all the hairs are glued in to hold them in place.

3. Rinse, brush facing down, under the running tap until the water runs clear. Then gently reshape it.

4. Place the handles of your brushes on a towel, trying to angle the heads face down off the edge of a flat surface, again ensuring no water is getting to where they're glued.

It's best to do this at night, that way your brushes will be dry and ready to go for the next morning.

Here's a list of my DO'S & DON'TS to keep your brushes in the best nick!

- **DON'T** throw your brushes loose into your handbag! I know we all do this, me included sometimes, but it's really bad for your brush hairs. They'll bend and break.

- **DO** carry them in a brush folio case (I use one from **Blank Canvas**). This is especially useful when travelling.

- **DON'T** leave your brushes to soak in a basin of water, the hairs will fall out if you do this. This is a mistake people often make, and then they wonder why the hairs are coming out.

- **DON'T** squash your brushes face down on a tissue or towel to clean them – you'll ruin them by doing this.

- **DON'T** overload your brush with too much liquid. Use a little, then add more if you have to.

- **DO** throw away any brush that is destroyed with foundation and can't be washed out. If you think it's gone beyond saving, don't waste your time, put it in the bin. Then buy a new one and take care of it.

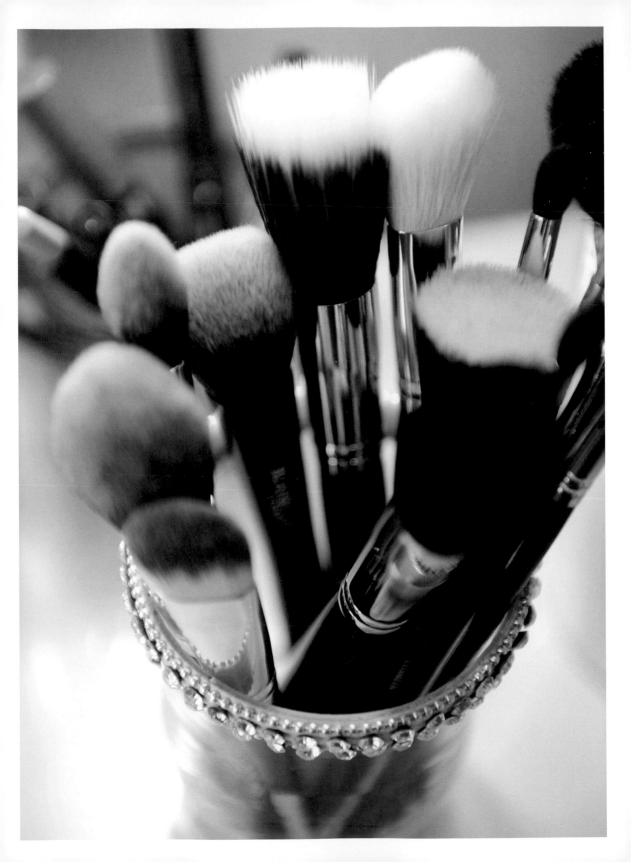

PERFECTING EYELINER

I love that eyeliner can define and change the shape of your eye in an instant! Liquid and gel eyeliners are definitely a little trickier than pencils but all it takes is some practice – and confidence!

Eyeliner is also something that everyone can wear, at any age and with any eye shape. Some women with hooded eyes (sometimes called 'bedroom eyes' as the lids tend to look a little heavy) think they can't wear liner, but they can! They perhaps just need to go for a thinner liner. Older women also think they can't get away with eyeliner but they absolutely can, and it can look really flattering to have more defined eyes that really stand out. Eyeliner isn't about just thick lines and a winged look (although we do cover that) – it can also create a more subtle, age-appropriate look.

When applying your eyeliner, it's best to do it after your eyeshadow and before your mascara. Here's how I do my eyeliner:

- If you're not confident using a liquid or gel product, go for a pencil – just make sure it isn't too pointy or hard. You may need to run it onto the back of your hand first.

- Starting from the outside in, draw tiny little lines all the way along your upper lash line. You don't need to draw one continuous line – take your time and then simply join them all up. I then like to get a very thin and fluffy eyeshadow brush, dip it into a brown or black eyeshadow and go over the liner. This will still give you the same effect and definition, it will just look smoked out.

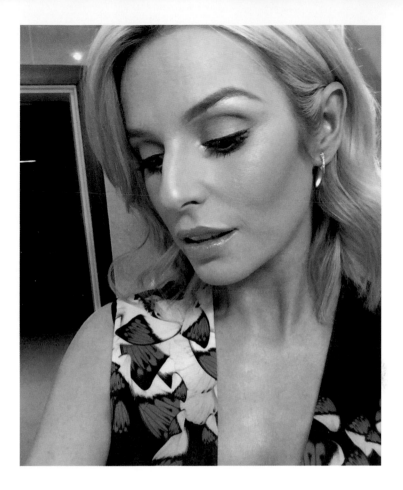

✳ **TIP** *Don't be afraid to stretch the skin a little with your other hand while you neaten everything up. Tip your head back as you are looking into the mirror – this will make your lids nice and flat as your eyes will be semi-closed, but you'll still be able to see what you're doing.*

If you need to clean up your edges to make the lines crisp, use a small angled or liner brush and dip it in some concealer and trace lightly along the edges.

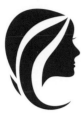

EXPERT TIP:
WINGED EYELINER

Expert Kate Rose Crean has provided some useful instructions on how you can achieve a perfect winged-eyeliner look:

1 Create a thin line from the inner corner of the eye to the outer corner using an angled brush and gel liner. Make sure the line is as close to the lashes as possible by using short feathery strokes.

2 Now place the angled brush just above the centre of the pupil and continue the line to the outer corner of the eye at an angle slightly higher than the original line. This will create your 'winged' effect.

3 Now connect both lines and fill in the gap in between.

4 For a longer wing like Pippa's, follow the angle from the bottom outer corner of your eye and elongate in one sweep outwards. The line should taper off to give a gorgeous feline shape.

5 Complete the look with lashings of mascara, beautiful skin and a soft nude lip.

Recommended products:
- **Inglot AMC eyeliner gel**
- **MAC 266 brush**
- **Charlotte Tilbury Full Fat Lashes**

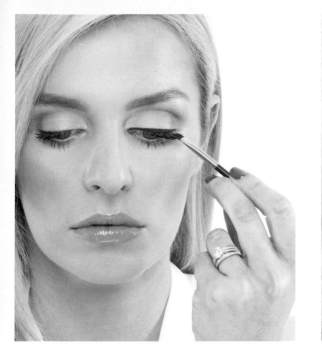

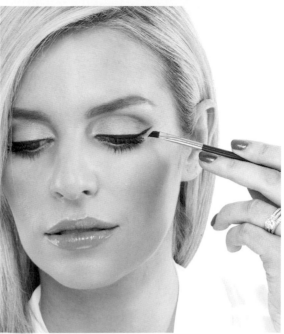

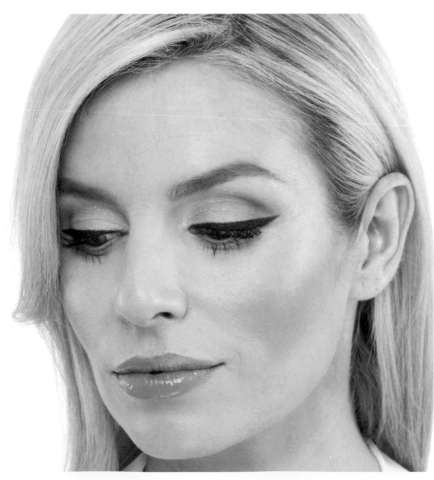

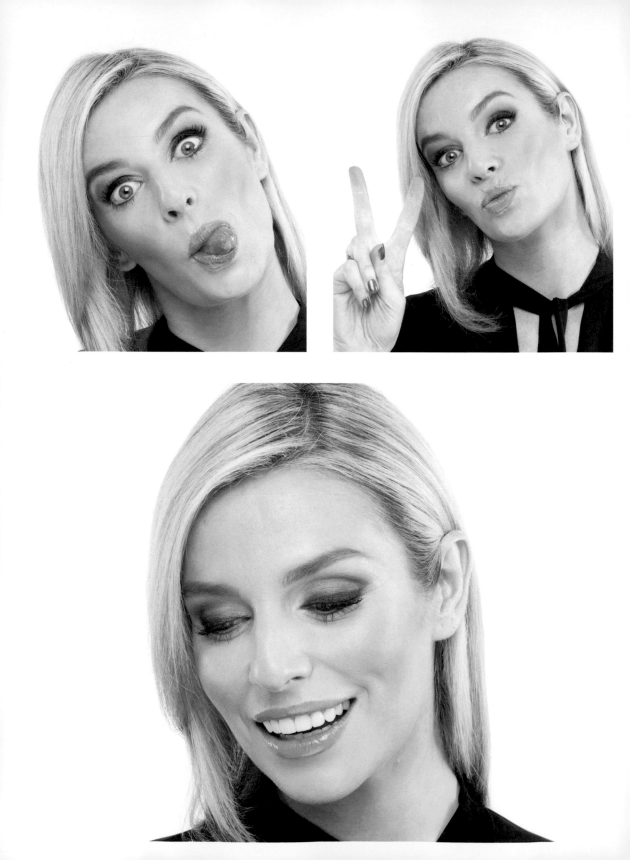

SMOKY EYE

A smoky eye is a dark, sultry look, which is great for a night out or party. There are literally hundreds of ways to achieve a smoky eye.

Colourwise, I like to use browns and cranberry colours to create my smoky eye. I might use a tiny bit of black in some areas, but I find using all black is very harsh and can be a little ageing.

1   Begin with a medium-sized flat eyeshadow brush to place your product. To start, I put a warm brown all over the lid and bring it up into my crease. Never go straight in using your darkest shade; you want to build it up.

2   Then, using your small fluffy blending brush, blend it all in, making sure you've no harsh lines in your crease. Good eye make-up is all about the blending!

3   Next, using your first brush (the medium-sized flat eyeshadow brush), take a darker shade, such as a cranberry, and repeat the first step all over again – place it all over the lids then blend, blend, blend!

4   Trace the upper lash line with a soft black pencil, then gently smudge with your small pointy eyeshadow brush.

✳   **TIP** *For a smoky eye in a flash, use just a soft, crayony eyeliner. Rim lids with a black pencil, making the line quite heavy; then smudge. You'll be left with a sexy sultry look in seconds.*

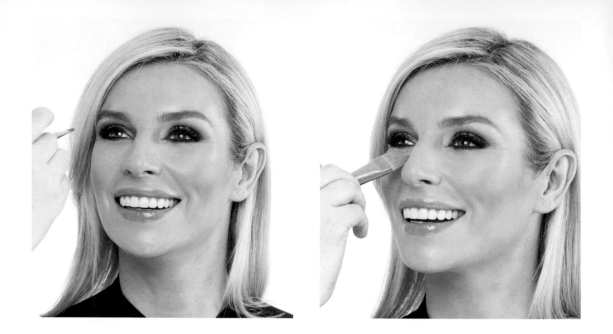

EXPERT TIP: FESTIVE EYES

I do love a bitta glitter! It's fun and festive and can jazz up any dark outfit. And you don't need to be twenty-one to glitter like a shimmery star, you just need not to go overboard with the application. Here's how to achieve that perfect festive look from make-up professional Kate Rose Crean.

1 Apply a cream base product, such as **Lancôme La Base Paupières Pro**, to your lid to give your eye make-up a little more staying power.

2 Line both your top and bottom lash line with **MAC Eye Kohl** pencil in Teddy, focusing more on the outer corners, and blend.

3 Using a **MAC 239 Eye Shader Brush**, apply a metallic shadow like **MAC Glitter in Gold** from lash to socket. For a more intense look, wet the brush and then pat the product onto the lid. Remember to place a little tissue underneath each eye to prevent fallout onto your skin!

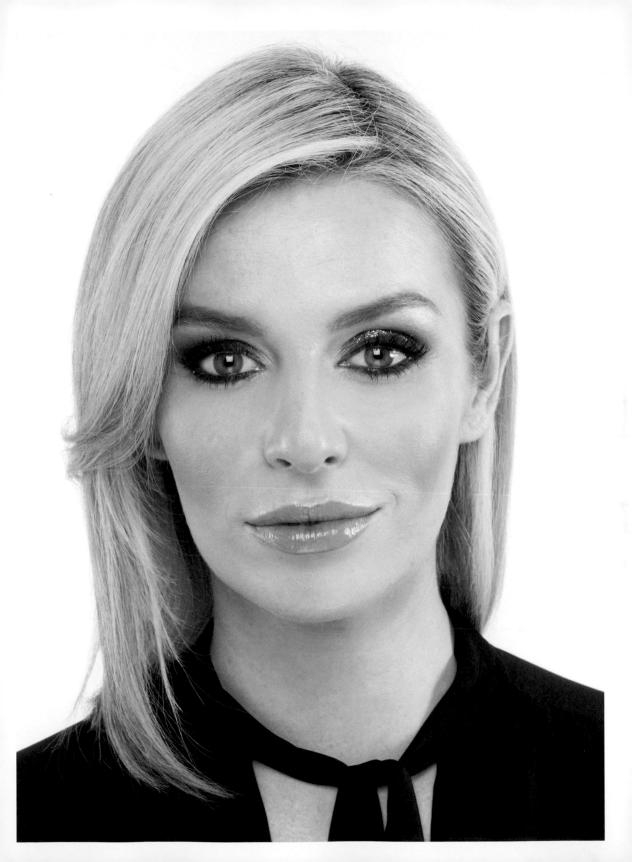

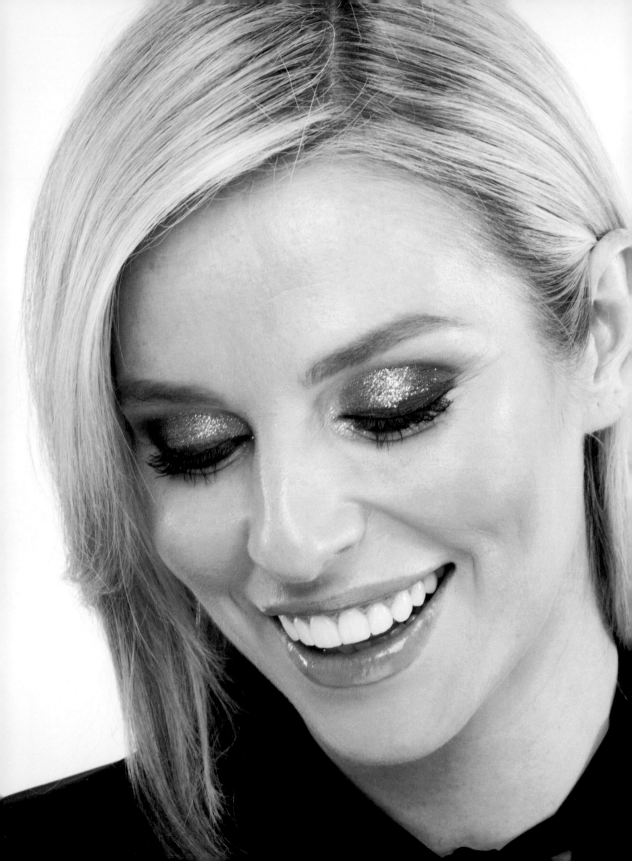

4 To darken the look, use a deep auburn brown eyeshadow and blend gently on the outer corners of your eye and through your bottom lash line, like I did with Pippa!

5 Curl lashes with **Shu Uemura's Famous Lash Curler** at the root, then middle and tip – this is fantastic for really opening up the eye!

6 Apply a generous coat of mascara to both upper and lower lashes for extra definition.

All shades of rich sumptuous metallics, like the one I used on Pippa, are perfect for lifting a winter complexion. For a more subtle look, brush a light wash of gold shimmer such as **MAC Paint Pot in Indianwood** across your lid and under your lower lashes, and leave out the liner.

Coppers and golds are gorgeous on blue eyes like Pippa's, mauves and slate greys work really beautifully on green eyes, while brown-eyed ladies are fortunate enough to be able to wear any colour and look amazing!

Other beautiful metallics to try out are:
- **Chanel Illusion D'Ombre – Epatant**
- **Laura Mercier – Black Karat**
- **Shiseido – Sable**

HOW TO ROCK RED LIPSTICK

Red lipstick is a universal classic and never goes out of style. Yet, many women assume they can't wear it – but they're wrong because everyone can rock a red lippy! The secret to red lipstick is finding the right shade for your skin tone and not going overboard with the rest of your make-up. Again, less is more!

The paler the skin, the bigger the pop. If you're going down the red lips route, you should stay light on the rest of your make-up or risk looking like a clown. Other things to note are:

- Red lipsticks tend to bleed, so always line your lips with a liner first. I find filling in the whole of my lips with the liner first creates a great base for the lipstick to hang onto.

- If I'm playing up my lips, I always go for a natural-looking eye, and vice versa – if my eyes are the feature, I'll go nude on my lips.

- A red lipstick with a blue undertone will suit most people. The blue undertones really make teeth appear whiter too. A great example of a lipstick like this is **MAC Ruby Woo.**

- If your complexion is pink, plum shades will flatter you. Women with yellow tones are flattered by warmer reds that have a brown base.

- Test them out! As with most make-up, it's all about trial and error and figuring out what suits you. There are so many different brands of lipstick, many of which are affordable, so if you're not sure what suits you or you're trying a new colour like red for the first time, buy some cheaper brands first.

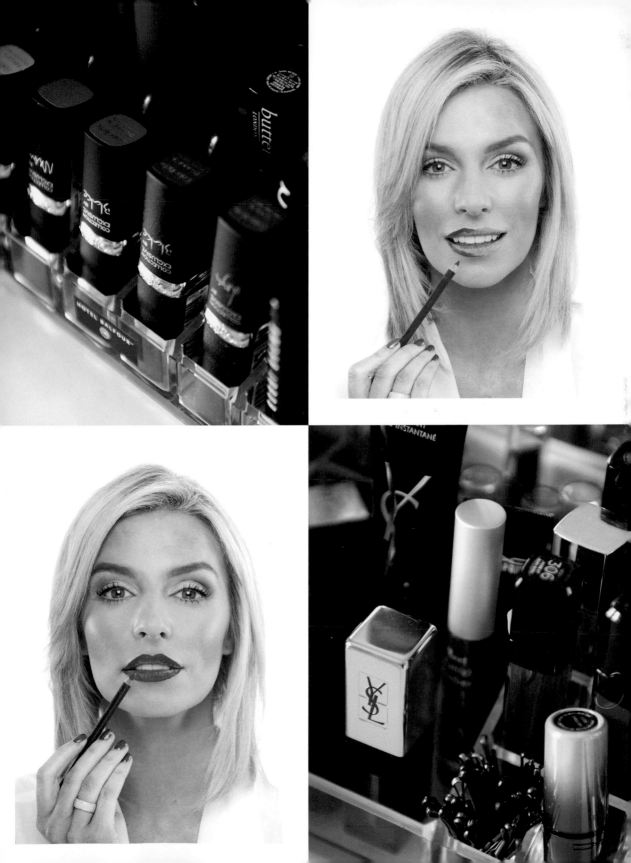

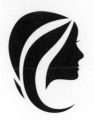

EXPERT TIP: RED LIPS

Here's how the make-up professional Kate Rose Crean creates the perfect red lips:

1 Begin by applying a good quality lip balm to the lips to keep them moisturized, then blot away the excess with a fine tissue. **Elizabeth Arden Eight Hour Lip Cream** is fantastic for soothing and smoothing.

2 Next, carefully outline and fill your lips with a lip liner. Lining your lips like this neutralizes their natural pinkness so that the lip colour you've chosen will be true to colour.

3 The easiest way to line your lips is to start at the highest point of your cupid's bow and follow your natural lip line to a corner of your mouth. Then repeat the same on the other side. Finish by lining your bottom lip in the same way.

4 Using a lip brush, apply your lipstick working from the middle of your lips out towards the edges. This gives you a clean, sharp shape. I love MAC brushes, and their retractable lip brush is perfect for fitting into your handbag. For Pippa, we went for a full-on statement lip look, but for a more stained finish, press the lip colour onto your lips with your finger. This softens and changes your lip shape, making it look less dramatic.

5   If you are going for a full-blown gorgeous red, then blot lips with a tissue and reapply another coat of lipstick. This will ensure that your lip colour will last for hours.

6   Finish off with a dab of highlighter to enhance your cupid's bow. This draws attention to the lip shape and really complements your lip colour.

Lip colours I love for this look are:
- **MAC Ruby Woo** – for a long-lasting matte blue/red lip finish
- **NARS Jungle Red** – not for the faint hearted! Its orangey/red tone is bright and eye-catching!
- **Rimmel Lasting Finish Kiss & Stay Lipgloss 500 Red Alert** – a gorgeous transparent berry red colour for a less dramatic look

 TIP *For warm complexions, choose cooler blueberry and plum shades. Cooler complexions suit richer reds with an orange or warm brown base.*

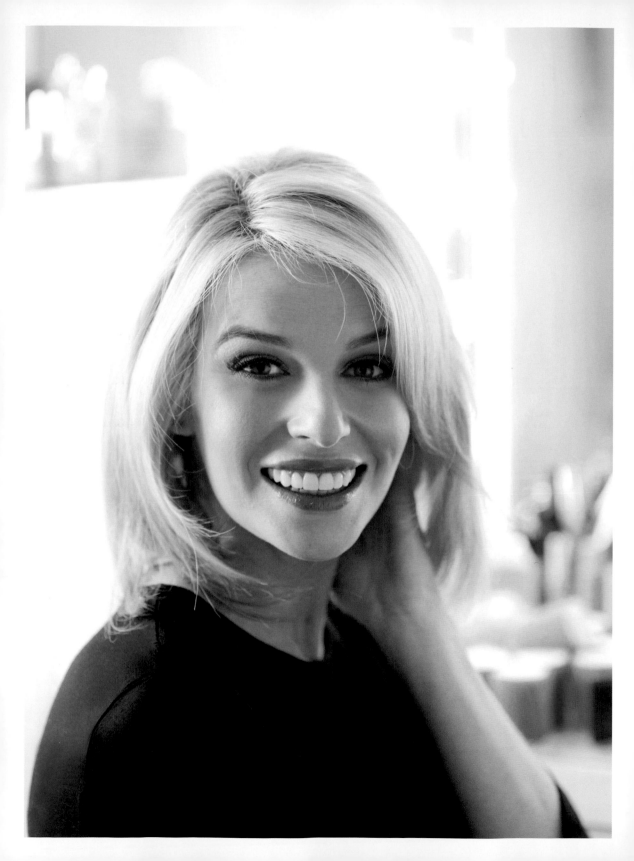

CHAPTER SIX

HAIR AND NAILS

A good haircut can transform your whole look and make you feel fantastic. Go for a style that suits the shape of your face as well as your lifestyle – remember you want to look good every day and not only when you've spent hours fussing over your locks. It's important also to look after your hair and scalp: try not to wash it too often as this strips your hair of its natural oils and be careful when you colour your hair or style it using heat as this can be really damaging.

There are also all sorts of things you can do to keep your hair looking shiny and healthy, from eating a healthy diet to using a hair mask – there are great products out there or just whizz up something simple at home (see pages 192–93).

Nails also finish off a look brilliantly. I like to get mine done once every two or three weeks – it's absolute bliss and such a relaxing thing to do. I recommend it! I go to nail supremo Michele Burke who has been an absolute godsend with my nails. Here she provides some expert tips and insider info on do-it-yourself manicures and how to keep your hands beautifully soft and supple.

HAIR

We all want shiny, healthy looking hair. And, if you're like me, you'll want to look like you have more of it too! Here are my top tips for making the most of your locks:

■ Don't wash your hair every day as this strips your hair of its natural oils. I have fine hair and I'm often really tempted to wash it everyday, especially when I wake up in the morning and look like Worzel Gummidge! My styles never seem to last well once I've slept on them but, still, I resist temptation and only wash it every other day. On Worzel-like days, I use a dry shampoo to give a bit of life and volume to my hair (I use **Redken Powder Refresh 01**), and I backcomb it and tie it up in a pony tail or loose bun.

■ Invest in a good hair dryer, the kind that you find in a salon. The more powerful, the better. Try to limit the use of straighteners and other styling tools that use heat – and when you are using them be sure to use a heat protectant first. My favourite is by **L'Oreal**.

■ Get your hair trimmed or cut on a regular basis. After I had Ollie, my hair was so long but lifeless-looking. I thought cutting it would be the worst thing to do to get it thicker and stronger-looking. Michael Doyle in Peter Mark also styles my hair, and he convinced me to go for a really fresh short cut. I did and I loved it. My hair has been in much better condition since.

■ If you're contemplating going for the chop, I say do it! A new haircut can transform not only the way you look but the way you feel. Never underestimate the power of an amazing cut. What if you don't like it? The good news is hair grows, so don't panic. And at least you'll have tried something different.

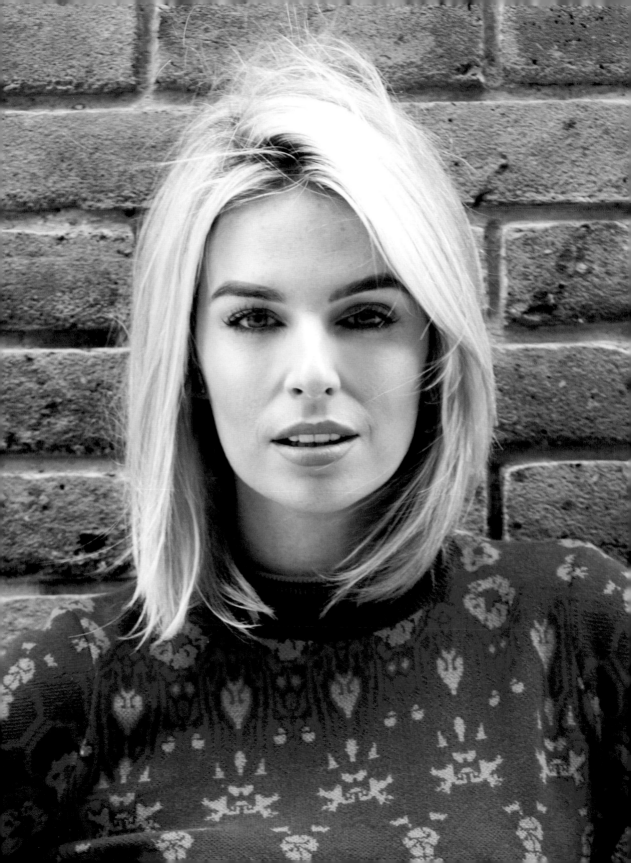

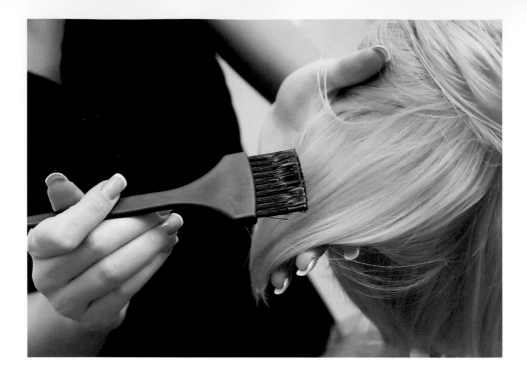

■   If you colour your hair, go to a good hair colourist, especially if you're blonde like me. It's important to get it right. Some of my friends with dark hair do it themselves and it looks amazing, but I could never do it myself. Oh my God, I've just gotten a flashback to my 'Sun In' days!! Remember that? My hair was orange!

I go to Peter Mark in Dublin. Terri Corbally colours my hair, she is fantastic. She listens and understands whatever I'm trying to get across. I have no idea what colours she uses to highlight my hair, she just does her thing after we have a chat. It's so important you trust your colourist's opinion and that they understand what you want. Be very clear and explain what you're thinking – bring photos for reference.

If it's your first visit to a new salon, tell them on the phone that you want a colour change as they'll more than likely get you in first to do a patch test on your skin to check the colour is suitable for you.

TIP *There are great products on the market that can hide any roots or greys in between salon visits. Some come in mini cans that you spray onto the root or there are others that you paint on. They wash out but they are just the job when you need something to tide you over. If you have dark hair, you can use an old mascara to paint onto your roots. My friend does this all the time and it works a treat.*

■ Eat your way to healthy hair. What we put into our bodies has a huge effect on our hair, its condition and its growth. So, eat a healthy diet that is low in sugar and refined carbs but high in healthy fats. Some of the best foods for healthy hair are eggs, fish, spinach, carrots, blueberries, chicken, sweet potatoes, lentils and walnuts.

■ Supplements can also help to maintain healthy hair and growth. Ask your pharmacy for advice on which ones would suit you, but in my experience you do have to take tablets for at least six months for them to work properly. So, be patient – they won't work in weeks.

■ Use hair masks once a week. If you don't want to spend much on a treatment, buy coconut oil from the supermarket, the one you cook with. It works wonderfully as a hair mask and you you can leave it on for as little or as long as you like. You can also make up some homemade hair masks, recipes are on the next page!

■ Protect your scalp. If you're in the sun, always wear a hat. Not only is this good for your hair colour, it will also prevent your scalp burning. Your scalp can also get sore when hair product builds up on your hair follicles, and this can lead to weak strands. Try squeezing a vitamin E capsule or some olive oil on to your hair, then give yourself a little head massage before rinsing throughly.

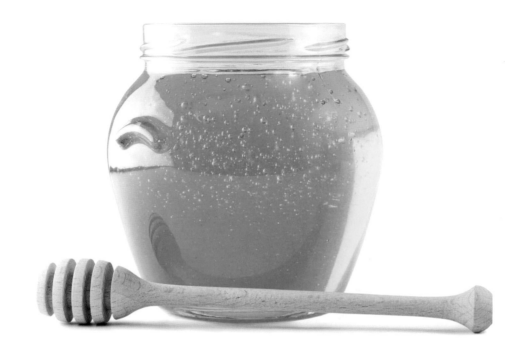

HAIR MASKS

Here are some simple hair masks you can make up at home.

Hydrating oil mask

1   Heat 4 tablespoons of **olive oil** in the microwave for 20 seconds.

2   Mix in 2 tablespoons of **honey**.

3   Apply to hair and leave it on for 20 minutes.

4   Rinse your hair.

Mask for shine

1   Mash 1 **avocado**.

2   Mix in ½ cup of **coconut milk** and 3 tablespoons of **olive oil**.

3   Heat everything in the microwave for 20 seconds.

4   Apply all over hair and leave on for 30 minutes.

5   Wash it all out.

Coconut oil mask

1   Mix 2 tablespoons of **coconut oil** and 1 tablespoon of **olive oil**.

2   Apply to hair, focusing on the ends.

3   Wrap hair into a bun and leave treatment on for 15–30 minutes.

4   Rinse, shampoo and condition hair.

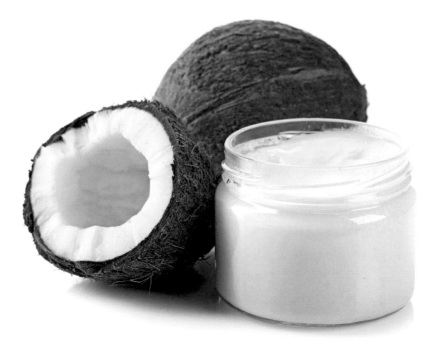

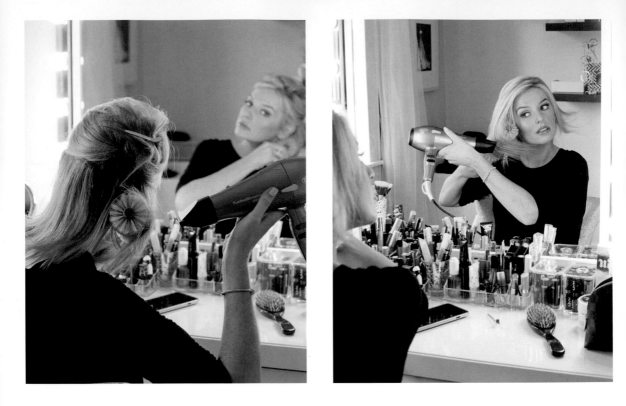

DIY WASH AND BLOW-DRY

I'm not an expert when it comes to hair, but I have learnt how to wash and blow-dry my hair pretty well – it just takes practice and a little bit of patience.

First, give your hair a good scrub, really lather up your shampoo of choice and scrub your scalp well. Do this twice, so your hair is really clean.

Conditioner is optional – we tend to pile on conditioner because we feel we need it when, actually, too much can just weigh down the hair, loading it up with product you don't need. So, less is more when it comes to conditioner in my opinion – only use it in areas where you need it and when you need it.

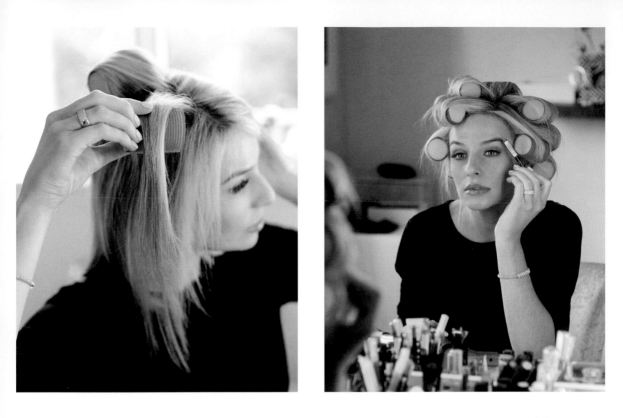

Gently towel-dry your hair. Now is when you can use a mousse to add volume, a serum or oil to smooth, or a treatment spray. I like **Redken One United Hair Treatment Spray** as it does about ten things in one: it detangles, protects from heat, adds shine, volume, smoothness, basically everything! I use this a lot and highly recommend it.

Then, I brush out my hair using a **Tangle Teezer** – these are fantastic and not only for kids' hair, but for your own, too, as they really detangle gently and quickly.

Now you're ready for the blow-dry. First, I blast my hair off using my fingers until my roots are practically dry.

Then I section my hair off – this step is important. I work from the bottom up, so I tie most of my hair up on top of my head leaving only the underneath section of my hair free.

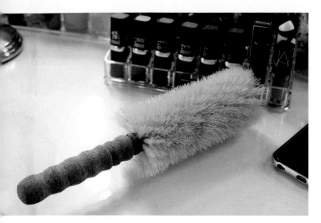

I get my big round wooden brush – I find the **Ibiza** brushes are the best brushes for hair styling. The wooden handles are so light and the big bristles are very soft on your hair. The bigger the barrel, the better here. I place my brush underneath a section of hair, place my hair dryer closely over the brush and hair (but not touching the hair) and pull my brush up and out, slightly turning my brush in towards my neck at the ends. I do this all around my head in small sections until I've worked my way to the top.

Now that most of my work is done I move onto my little secret weapons – something I was taught by my mother – velcro rollers. These are the best things you could ever have when styling your hair. Every day, my mum would have her velcros in while doing her make-up. Now I know why! They give the best lift and volume. I use the medium-sized ones – the smaller the velcro the tighter the slight wave it will create, so I like to use the fatter ones as I just want them for volume at the root.

Starting at the top of my head, I put my rollers in all over and leave for at least thirty minutes while I do my make-up or get dressed. Then, I gently take them out and use a comb to style and brush my hair into place.

Finish with a light spray of **L'Oreal Elnett**. Again, this is something else that reminds me of my mother – she was forever spraying Elnett!

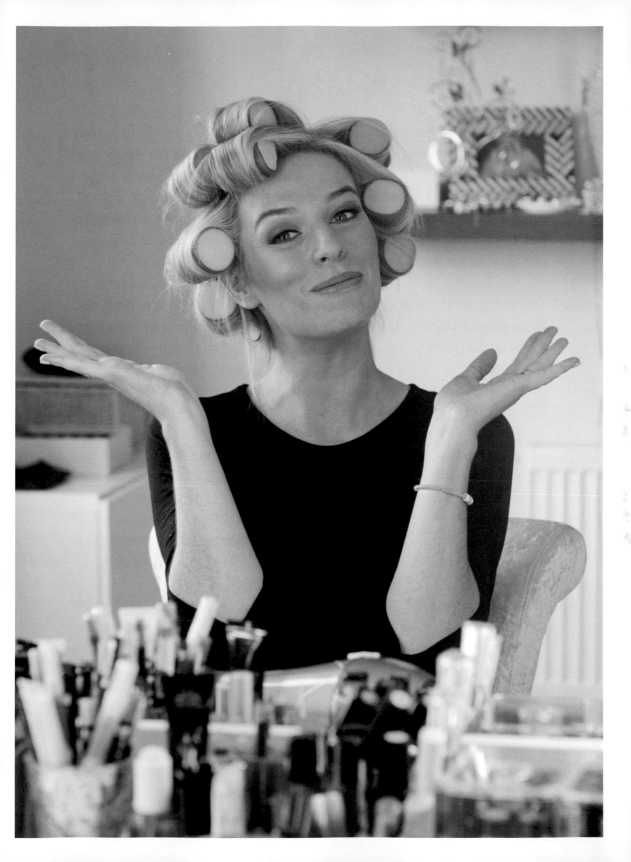

NAILS

For years, my worst habit without a doubt was biting my nails – they were little stubs and I hated them. They constantly felt weak and brittle, so I just bit them off. I tried all of those nail hardeners and yucky tasting topcoats to stop me biting them but nothing worked. Then I moved onto getting false tips – I kept that up for a few years but once I become a mum it just seemed too impractical and time consuming for me to keep up.

Then I found Michelle – my little nail saving fairy! She got my nails into presentable shape for the first time ever. She gave me a proper manicure, filed my nails to a short length and applied a **Gelish** polish – which was the only thing I wasn't tempted to bite through. Michelle kept them short until they became healthy and stronger. They're still short, which is the style I like, but they certainly aren't stubby like before!

Going to get my nails done every two to three weeks is a treat just for me. Gelish polish is my favourite as it's the most durable. I love its high glossy finish, it never dulls and doesn't chip on me. Between salon visits, I try to be good at home by applying hand cream daily and cuticle oil most evenings too. I keep these by my bed as I'm more likely to reach for them in the evenings.

To give youself a really nice treat at home, give your hands a scrub using Michelle's homemade hand scrub (see recipe on page 205) followed by lathering your hands in a nice cream. My favourite is by **Clarins** – it's a hand and nail treatment but also fantastic for keeping age spots at bay. You could also wear hand mittens overnight, which will help the cream to really soak in. You can do this on your feet too! Apart from waking up with baby soft hands and feet, your other half will get a great laugh at the sight of you! Mine does anyway!

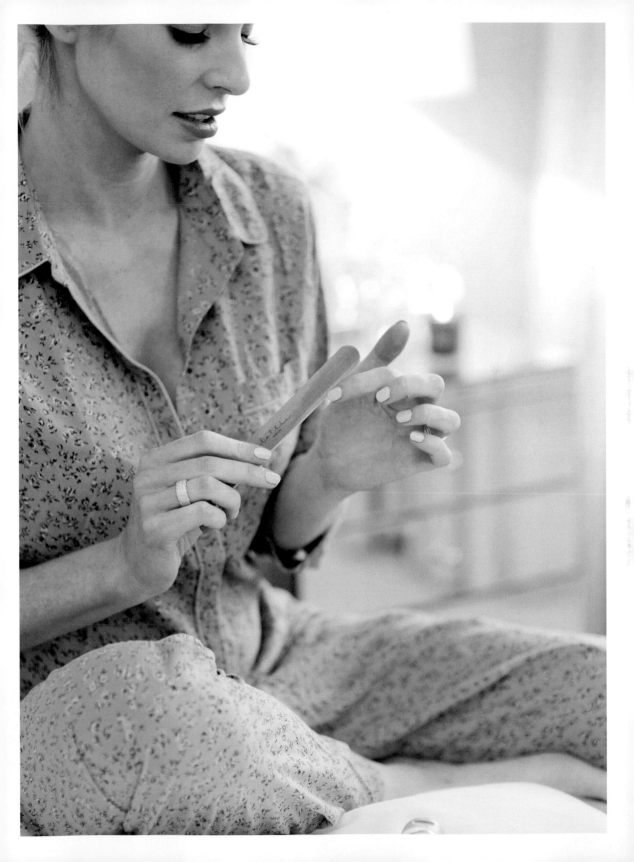

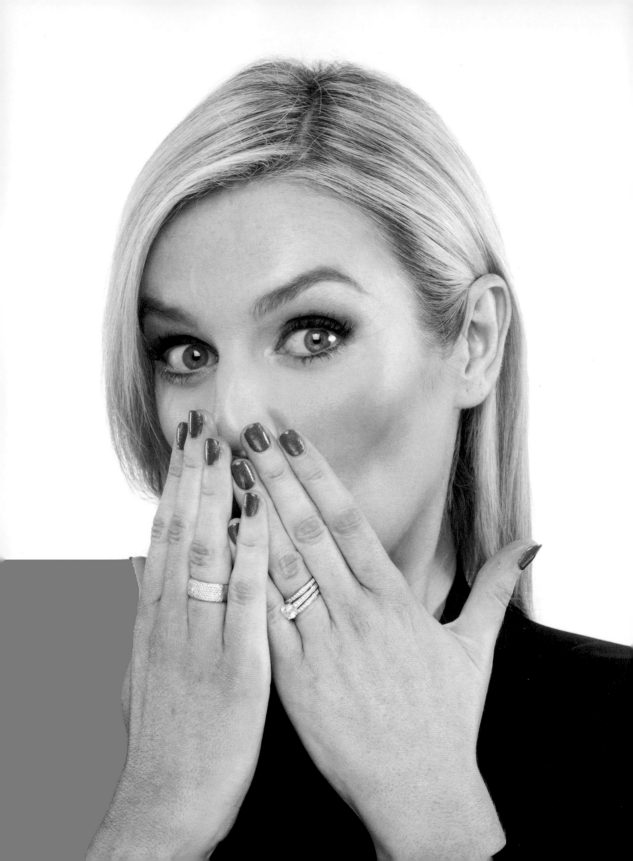

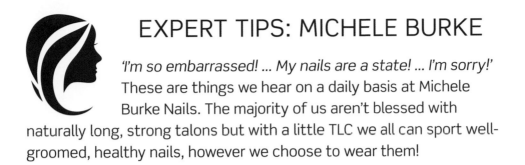

EXPERT TIPS: MICHELE BURKE

'I'm so embarrassed! ... My nails are a state! ... I'm sorry!'
These are things we hear on a daily basis at Michele
Burke Nails. The majority of us aren't blessed with
naturally long, strong talons but with a little TLC we all can sport well-
groomed, healthy nails, however we choose to wear them!

What kind of nail style are you after? Are you a ...

High maintenance chick
You like to wear a long claw-like manicure, preferably of the acrylic/
gel variety. You love to adorn your nails with jewels, glitter and the
hottest colours for the season. You always keep on top of the
latest trends.

Speed queen
Having your nails done is an essential part of your beauty routine.
You love to be in and out of the salon as fast and polished as possible.
A super strong, shiny three-week manicure is your style of choice;
a brand like **Gelish** is perfect for your busy lifestyle.

DIY dame
A salon visit is a treat! You like to pop in for a nail treatment in
preparation for special occasions and holidays. Otherwise mani
maintenance is all on you.

Whatever category you're in, here are some essential maintenance
tips to keep your hands and nails looking fresh and youthful.

The rules of hand and nail care

Housework, as painfully boring as it is, has to be done! Rubber gloves are essential to keep chemicals like bleach away from the skin. Cleaning products can wreak havoc on the skin, leaving it dry, cracked and irritated.

A natural cuticle oil and hand cream should be used daily. Preferably every time the hands are washed. If that feels like too much maintenance, apply your lotions and potions at nighttime. The skin repairs itself while we sleep, so give it a helping hand to heal and moisturize, moisturize, moisturize! For maximum absorption of products, pop on a pair of soft white cotton gloves afterwards.

Coconut oil is a dream product for its super moisturizing, antioxidant and anti-ageing properties. We are also big fans of **Hand & Nail Harmony Nourish Cuticle Oil**, which contains a unique blend of grapeseed oil, kukui nut oil, sesame and vitamin E to keep cuticles and nails in super condition.

Don't pick or bite at the nails, enhancements or gel polish. Having regular manicures, following the correct home care routine and returning to the salon for professional product removal will guarantee you fabulous fingertips ready to flaunt!

DIY Manicure

For my DIY dames, follow these steps to create a long-lasting, chip-free, salon-quality manicure.

1 Shape the free edge of nail with a soft, smooth nail file – no emery boards allowed as these can split the edges if the nail is weak.

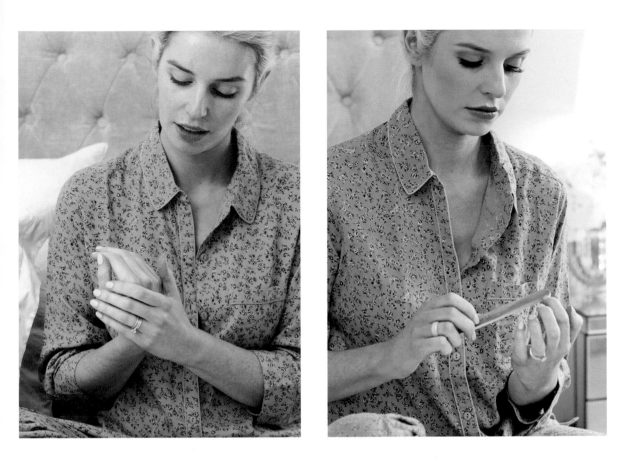

2 Prep the nails. Push back the cuticles with a metal cuticle pusher (these can be sanitized) or an orangewood stick that can be binned after use. A good time to do this is straight after a bath or shower as the skin will be softer and easier to work with.

Use a three-way buffer, which has three different file strength sections to buff the nail plate. This is like an exfoliation for the nail. Buffing is essential for removing any dry, flaky edges and ensuring long lasting polish wear.

Wipe over the nail with nail polish remover to remove any dust and oils.

3 Apply a base coat, ALWAYS! A base coat is like a primer for a perfect polish application. There are many different types, from ridge fillers to strengthening. A base coat also protects the nails from staining.

4 Apply two or three thin coats of your preferred brand and colour polish. Painting each coat as thinly as possible is important, to help the drying process and the all-over look of the finished manicure. No one wants to see lumpy bumpy nail polish. I love to work with the **Morgan Taylor** brand of polish. These are salon-quality nail lacquers that have a huge colour range of super pigmented polishes, which are long lasting and affordable.

5 Top coat all the way. This layer seals in all the other layers applied and prevents the chipping of the polish. The finish of a top coat can be fast drying, matte or super shiny. Choose this to match how you're feeling on the day!

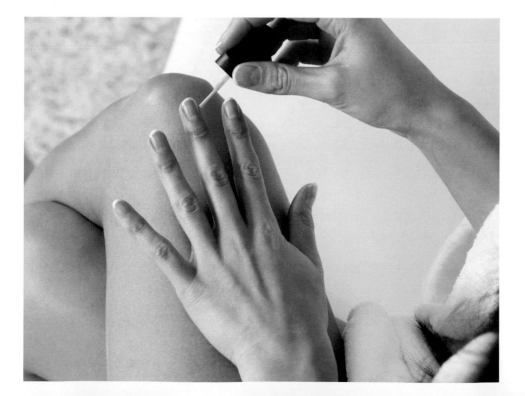

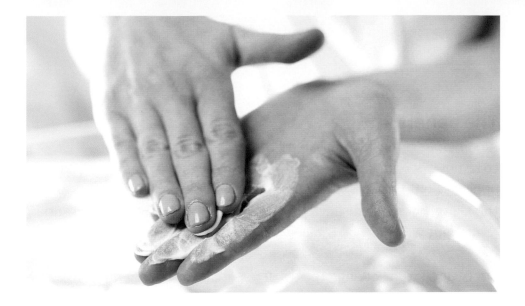

PERFECT PAWS

At Michele Burke Nails, we're all about giving nature a helping hand, and there's something very satisfying about making your own homemade anti-ageing hand scrub (which can be used on the body too!).

Tropical anti-ageing exfoliator

Ingredients
- 4 tablespoons brown sugar
- 4 tablespoons sea salt
- 1 tablespoon coconut oil
- 1 tablespoon fresh lemon juice (grate the peel too, if you fancy!)
- 1 tablespoon honey

Method
- Mix all the ingredients into a smooth paste.
- Soak hands in warm water to soften the skin.
- Gently massage the scrub onto damp skin for 2–3 mins to gently exfoliate skin.
- Rinse off, towel dry and moisturize.

The benefits

A homemade sugar scrub like this creates a gentle abrasion to remove accumulated dead skin cells. The gentle massaging application technique of the scrub also enhances blood circulation to the skin. This increases collagen production and skin cell regeneration to prevent wrinkles and other signs of ageing.

Coconut oil won't change the pH of your skin, so it's not irritating. It contains antioxidants that help diminish fine lines, and is a great natural moisturizer.

Lemon juice is a natural exfoliant; the citric acid acts as a gentle 'skin peel' removing the superficial top layer of dead skin cells. This will result in smooth skin when used regularly. Lemon juice can also brighten and lighten the skin helping to diminish pigmentation such as age spots.

Honey is full of antioxidants, which are great for slowing down the appearance of ageing. It is extremely moisturizing and soothing, boosting the complexion and helping to create a youthful glow. AMAZING!

Remember ladies, ageing is out of your control; how you handle it, though, is in your hands. It's never too early to start your anti-ageing manicure routine!

Michele x

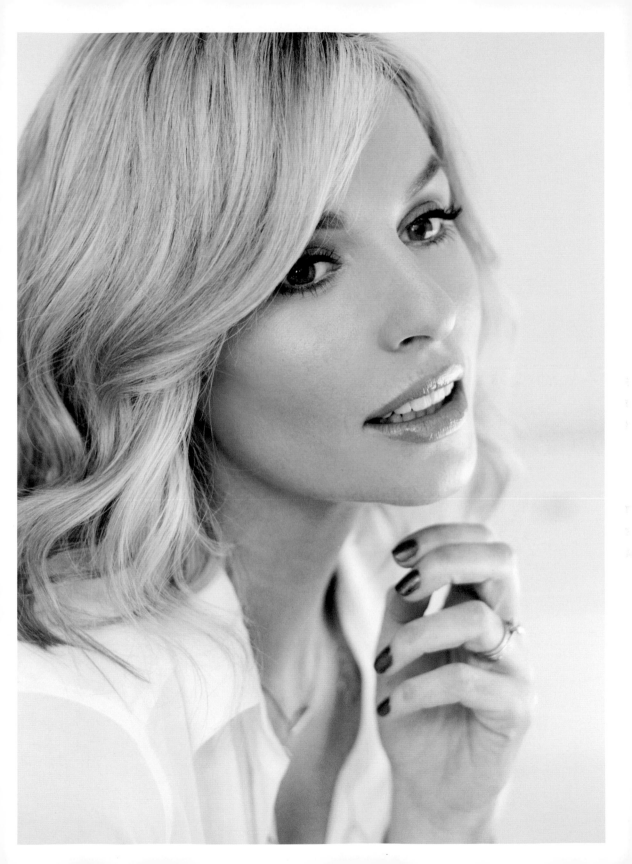

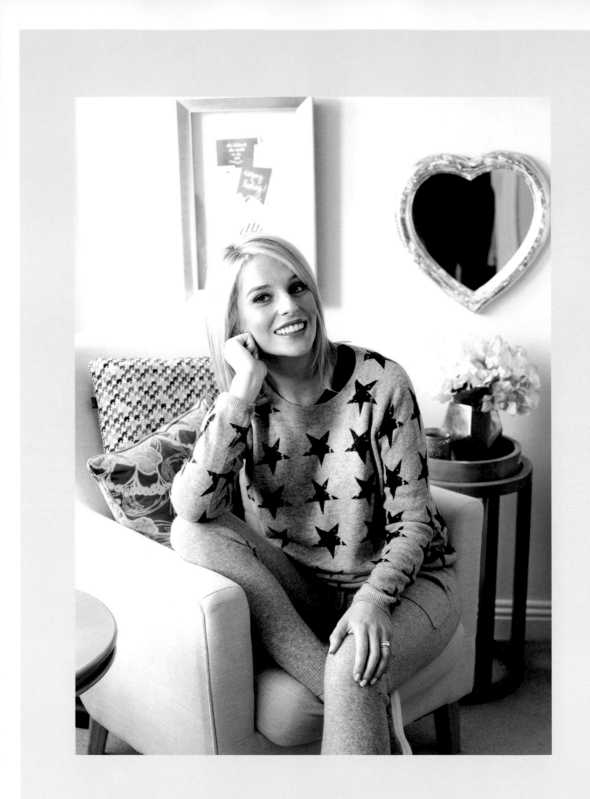

For what it's worth:
It's never too late to
be whoever you want
to be. I hope you live
a life you're proud of,
and if you find that
you're not, I hope you
have the strength to
start over.

F. Scott Fitzgerald

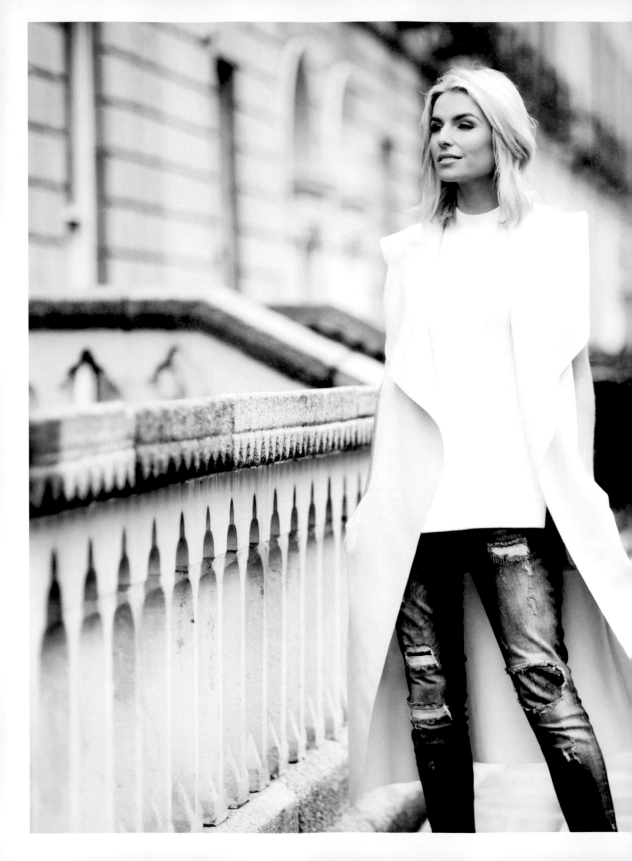

PART THREE: LIFESTYLE

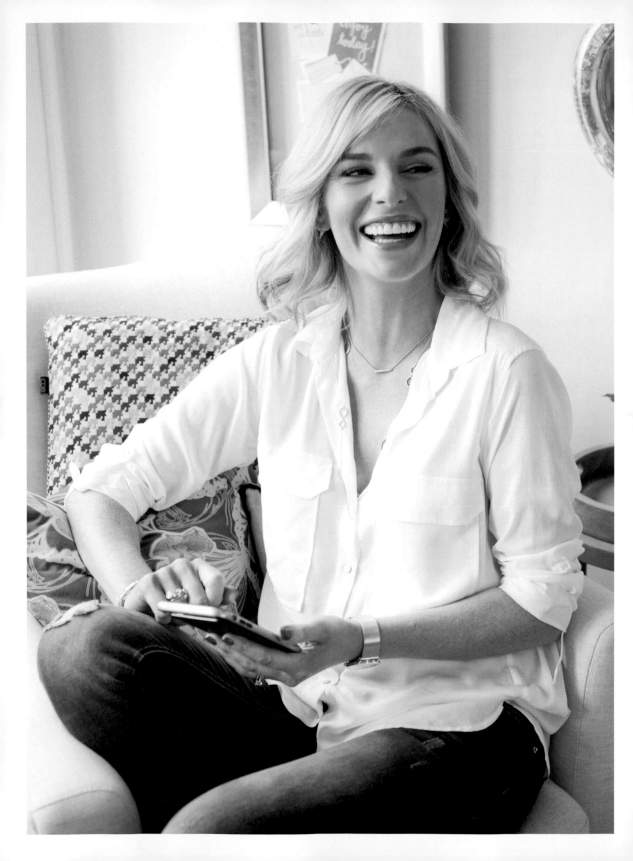

CHAPTER SEVEN

STYLE YOUR HOME

I love our home and I love decorating it. Years ago, confessing you liked DIY or fixing up your house was a sure sign that you were getting older and that your youth was firmly behind you. But nowadays all ages are into interiors – even my teenage stepdaughter loves her dressing table and doing up her bedroom.

I've always had a passion for interiors, something else I have inherited from my mum. She had such a creative eye, and the ability to make a room look amazing without spending much money. For me, taking pride in your home and making it a cosy and comfortable sanctuary for your family is so important.

Just a few simple touches can make all the difference to a room, from a beautiful throw to the warm glow of a pillar candle and a well-positioned mirror. Storage is a big one, as clutter can add to my stress levels, so I really try to organize my stuff, especially all my beauty products and shoes, which, as you can imagine, can really pile up!

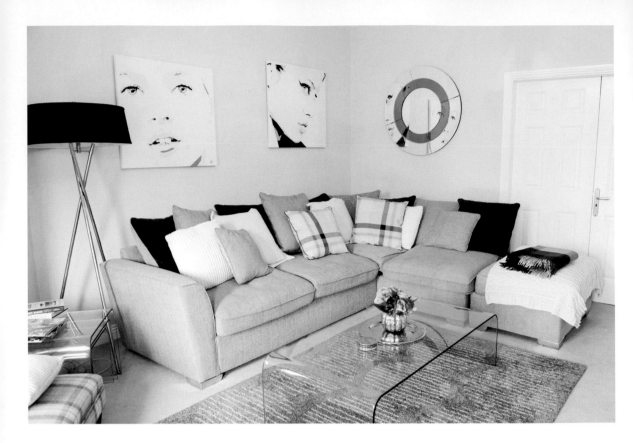

Since I met my husband, we've lived in four houses. Moving home is a bit of a trial and the last one was the worst as we had more furniture than ever before, plus a whole new person to bring along too – who knew a baby could accumulate so much stuff?! So, I'm really used to packing up and unpacking, and at least the process helps you to declutter and get rid of anything you don't need.

The house we're in now is beautiful, but it's not our 'forever house'. We plan on moving one last time (in a few years) and that'll be it. Forever!

I've spent the first year here making it our own and decorating it to our liking. As it's not our forever home, we haven't spent a fortune on it and I think that's the tricky part – doing things cost-effectively but in a way that looks much more expensive than it actually is.

For me, taking pride in your home and making it a cosy and comfortable sanctuary for your family is so important.

LIVING ROOM

Whatever your taste in interiors, I always think a living room should look inviting, cosy and elegant – a room that you can't wait to get home to on a Friday evening after work to relax and put your feet up. When you're entertaining, it can also be somewhere where your guests will feel at home and relaxed.

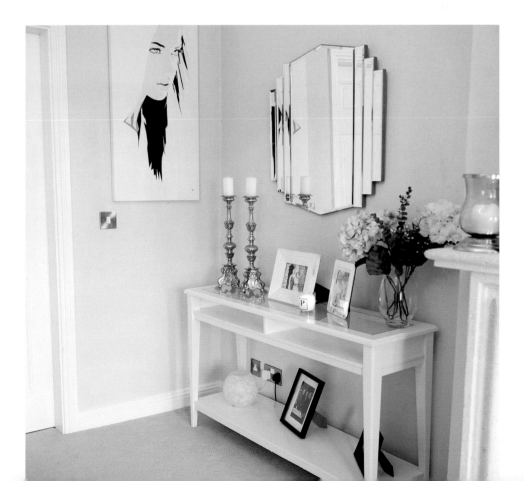

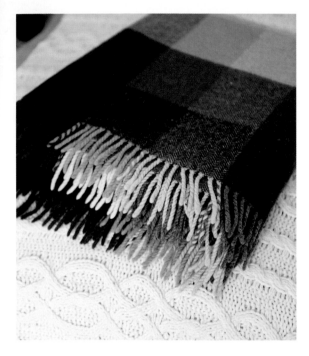
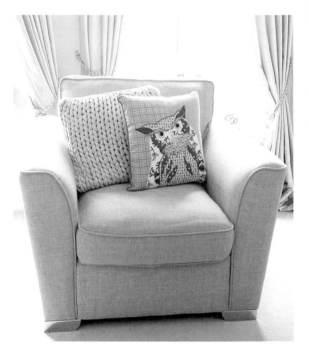

COLOURS

Neutral colours are always a top choice for me. Whites, creams and greys are what I go for when it comes to living rooms. Neutral colours make your home appear cleaner and more spacious. They also help to create more light, which is always a good thing.

If you love colour, by all means go for it and don't be afraid. A really bright and colourful abstract painting in a room can be so eye-catching and beautiful. Pick colours out of it and get some cushions or a rug in similar colours . Keep to a colour theme, though, and don't go overboard as that's when things begin to clash and look busy – unless that's the kind of look you love!

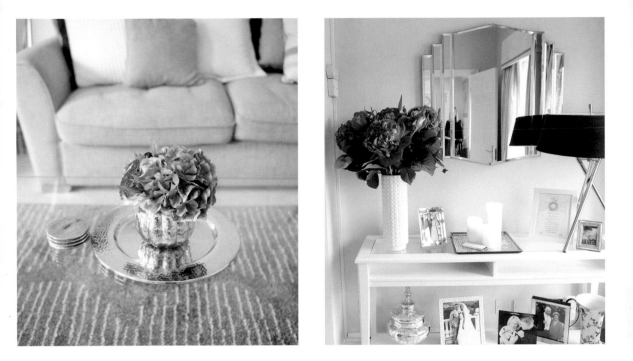

When choosing paint colours for your living room, take your time and always test them out. Paint invariably looks different on the wall to how it appears on a chart. The finished effect also depends on the size of your room, how much light is coming in and what you have in it.

I have various rooms in our house painted the same colour, yet the walls look different in each one.

So it's very important to test your options – most paints come in tester pot size – and live with them on the wall for a couple of days.

SIMPLE TOUCHES

A few years ago, we invested in a beautiful L-shaped couch and it's looked great in each house we've had because it's in a neutral light grey colour. When you have a neutral couch or chair it's easy to add just a few touches for a different look. At Christmas, I'll add red and festive cushions, then once spring arrives, I'll throw on some fresh cushions with hints of yellow and duck-egg blue. I'll do the same with throws – I have a few different ones depending on the season. This works really well and can change the entire aesthetic of the room. I have a friend who alternates her curtains twice a year too – I haven't done that myself, but it's a good idea as it completely transforms the look of the room.

I'm also a sucker for a really lovely coffee table in a living room. I like them to be low and uncluttered, with maybe just some candles as your centrepiece or a flower display. If you're putting candles on your table, use an uneven number – maybe three or five – it just looks better and anything arranged in odd numbers seems to be more appealing and memorable!

Candles also look good displayed on a tray of some sort – either a square or circular mirrored tray adds simple sophistication.

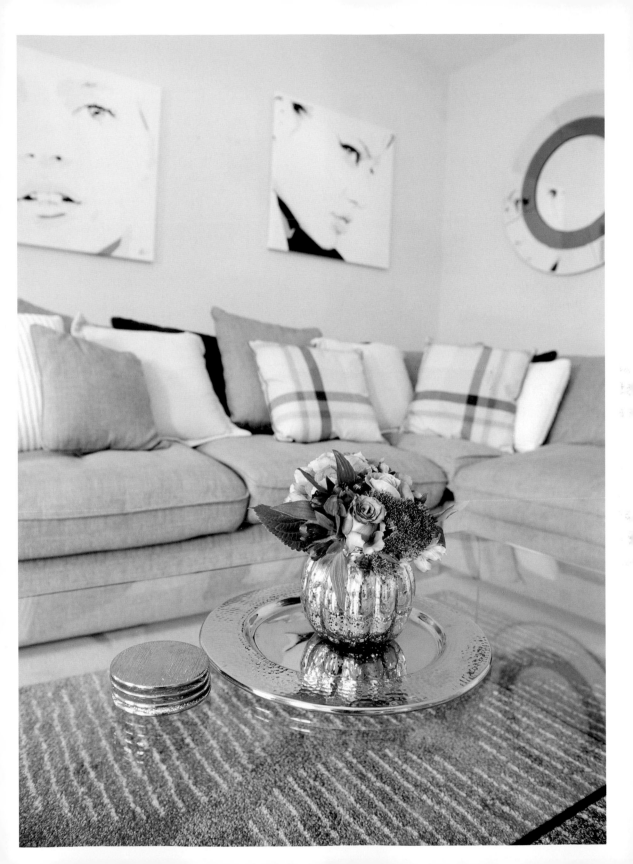

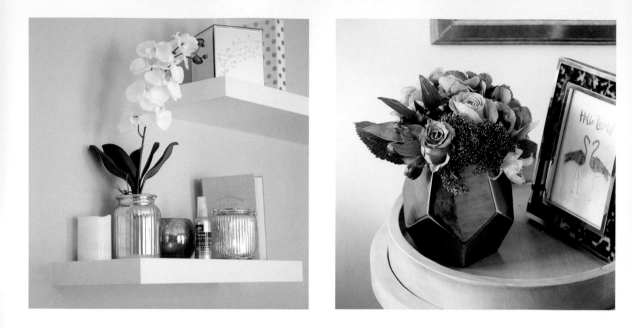

FLOWER POWER

Flowers can make a real impact in a room – a beautiful flower display is sometimes all you need to create that 'wow' factor. Everyone will comment on them. And if your room is neutral, the pop of colour from flowers is so uplifting.

I adore pink or white flowers with hints of green. My favourite flowers are peonies, roses and hydrangeas, which will always remind me of our wedding. We had white hydrangeas everywhere, they were so stunning. In the springtime, I adore tulips. A bunch of bright tulips in a kitchen is magnificent and you can simply use big glass candle holders or jam jars to display them. In any living room, white tulips are so calming and elegant. In a hall, I love tall displays of white lillies.

It's always lovely to be given flowers, but I also make sure not just to wait until then. I usually buy myself fresh flowers once a week, on a Friday or Saturday. It's a lovely treat and a cheap way of cheering yourself up. Try it!

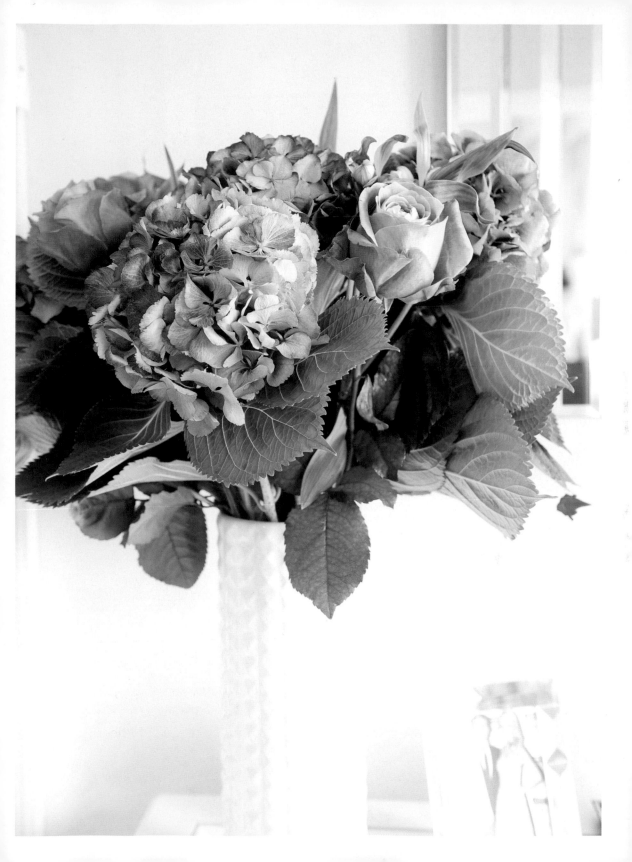

CANDLES

I have a serious love for candles. If you ever want to buy me a gift, you can't go wrong with a candle – just saying! If you come into our house or my office, day or night, I'll have candles burning. To me, they make the room look warm and inviting, and there's nothing nicer than the smell of a beautifully scented candle filling the house.

Like so many things, I must have inherited my love of candles from my mum. However, she took it to another level as I remember growing up she would have real candles on our Christmas tree. Yes, you read that correctly! Can you imagine how dangerous that was? We're lucky the place never went up in flames! I think the tradition was very common before the invention of Christmas tree lights but less common in the 1980s when I was a child.

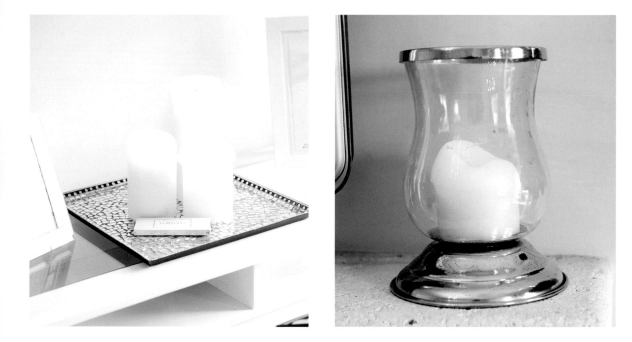

There are so many different ways candles can be used to create a warm atmosphere. I love large pillar candles in hurricane lamps by the fireplace or, if you have an open fire that you're not using, try replacing a roaring fire with large candles – it'll create a stylish focal point for your living room.

With really good quality scented candles like Jo Malone, don't be tempted to burn them for too long – you'll only waste them. They actually only need about 30 minutes to scent a room.

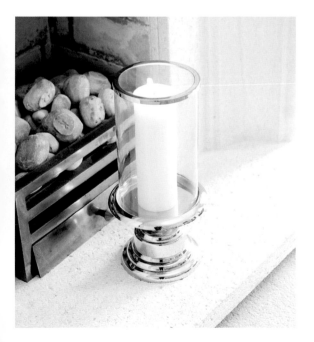

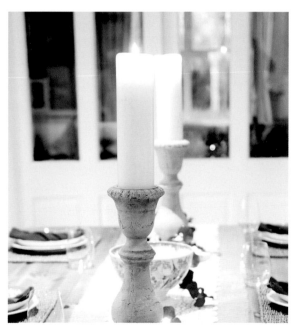

If you're worried about the potential fire hazard of using candles, or spilt wax, you can always use battery operated candles. I have ones with timers, which is very handy as it saves you turning them on and off manually. The battery operated ones are a much safer option in general if you've got small children around. I also like to use them on my bookshelf in our bedroom as they create a lovely relaxing atmosphere.

My favourite candles to burn are **Jo Malone** – I adore **Pomegranate Noir**. I was given the room spray recently and that, teamed with the candle, is absolutely gorgeous. Everyone comments on it when they walk into our house.

 TIP *If you have a large candle in a jar or glass holder that's burnt out – something like a Yankee candle – clean it out by filling it with nearly boiling water. (It's best to wear rubber gloves when you do this.) The wax will easily come away with the water and a little bit of a scrub.*

MAKE THE MOST OF YOUR SPACE

When it comes to the look of my house, I prefer the minimal, uncluttered look, mainly because I think it helps to make rooms feel bigger and brighter. One thing my mum wasn't good at was decluttering. Everything had a place alright, but she just had so much of it – books, ornaments, you name it.

When decorating any small room in the house, create a focal point – one area or feature that will draw the eye. In the dining room, this will probably be the table. In the bedroom, it will most likely be the bed. Make that focal point the star of the room. Arrange the furniture so that focus is drawn to that area, and keep the décor in the rest of the room to a minimum – limit the number of accessories. You might want the odd candle or pot of flowers, but don't go overboard with these as it will make your room feel cluttered and smaller.

Sometimes, the most effective way to increase usable space is simply to reorganize the furniture. Remove all clutter, and leave just two or three types of accessories, such as magazines displayed on an end table, vases, throws or pillows. It helps also to take items off the floor, such as stereo equipment, vases with dried flowers or potted plants, and reposition them on shelves and pieces of furniture instead. You'll be amazed the difference that makes alone.

Be clever with the space you have. A corner entertainment centre, TV cabinet or, better yet, a flat screen TV mounted on the wall provides more space and opens up the room. Make the most of any built-in cupboards, shelves or alcoves to maintain a decluttered look.

One of the best and least expensive ways to decorate a small room and create the illusion of space is to use a mirror. I love mirrors and have them in nearly every room – not to check myself out(!) but because they make such an impact. A large mirror on the long wall of a narrow room will make the room appear much wider. A decorative mirror, especially a large wall mirror, will give the illusion of space when strategically placed to reflect light or an attractive element in the room, such as a window with a scenic view, a doorway into another room, a fireplace or an artwork.

For a clean, uncluttered look, another good tip is to avoid covering your walls with lots of pictures. One large painting works better than a group of small paintings, and if you do decide to go for smaller pictures, put them on just one feature wall, rather than all the walls in the room.

I know how hard it is to keep things minimal-looking and decluttered when you have kids. Before we had a separate playroom, our sitting room was taken over every day by toys. Each night, I'd spend an hour putting everything back into units and buckets. So, when we moved into our current house, straight away I knew I wanted a separate room for toys and playing. Our sitting room has adjoining doors into a dining room, and my husband and I agreed we'd get better use out of it if we turned the dining room into a playroom, so that's what we did. It's been the best decision ever!

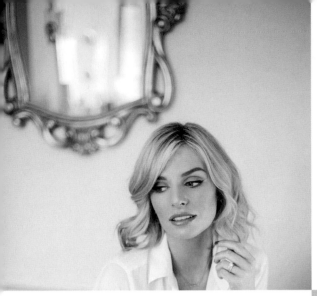
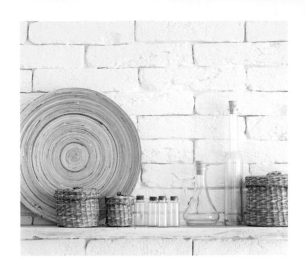
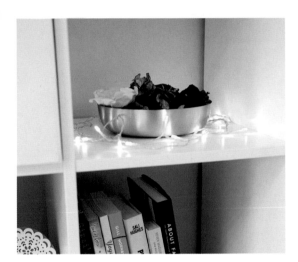
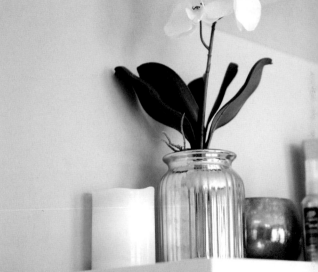
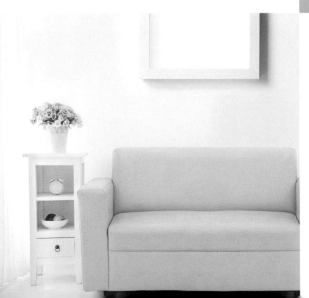
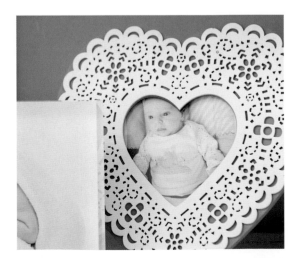

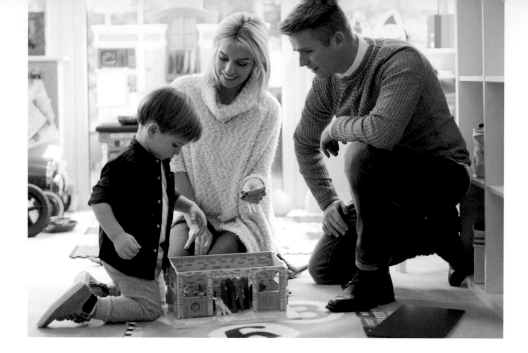

PLAYROOM

My son Ollie is three now, and like most little boys and girls he has accumulated lots of toys over the years with birthdays, Christmas and everything in between. He could open his own toyshop if he wanted! He's had stages of having way too many toys, so now I make an effort to do regular clear outs. This way he can clearly see what he has and can actually play with them instead of being overwhelmed by all the mess and clutter.

All mothers have those 'we-can't-live-this-way-anymore' moments, when you wish you could just bin everything. So what's the answer? The bad news is that kids and clutter go hand-in-hand. But the good news is that you can control the clutter. Set aside an afternoon and start making a plan. If your child is old enough, they can definitely be involved. Adding a sense of fun, or playing games, while you clear up, will help. Let the child be the decision-maker as much as possible so that they will take ownership of the newly organized and clutter-free room.

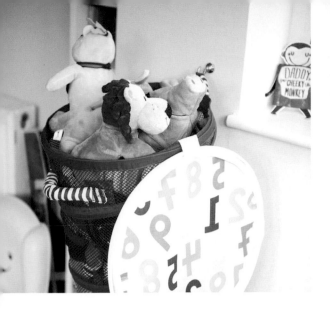
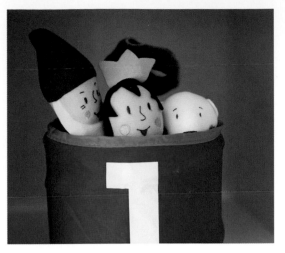

The first step is to gather some bins, bags or boxes and label them as follows:

Bin
Some toys are just beyond repair, so if this is the case bin them.

Give away or sell
Another mother or child will be delighted with your unwanted toys. You could donate them to a local playgroup, charity or school, or give them to your friends.

Store
Kids grow out of toys quickly but you can store anything you want to keep for younger siblings, family or just in case! I like to store toys away in big clear boxes and mark them according to age, for example 0–6 months.

Repair
Some toys or animals just need a good clean or some TLC and can be brought back to life.

STORAGE

For storing and displaying toys we bought a big unit in IKEA. I buy a lot from IKEA simply because it's affordable and practical. This box unit is perfect for displaying the toys, again because Ollie can see where things are.

If you're using drawers in a unit, it's a good idea to label what's in the drawers. This will teach your kids where things go and hopefully they'll be inclined to put them back in their place!

I also have lots of colourful plastic buckets and soft containers and will keep farm animals in one, dinosaurs in another, and horses in another. Ollie's obsessed with small animals he can carry around. Lego goes into another bucket, and so on.

We also have a little kitchen in Ollie's playroom. He really loves this and gets lots of use out of it. He often makes me dinner and cups of tea. Hopefully, he'll keep that up when he's older and do it for real – I won't hold my breath! Any cousins or friends of Ollie's that come over love it too – it's a big hit!

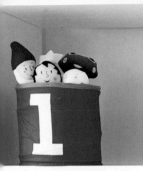
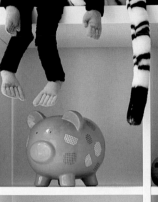
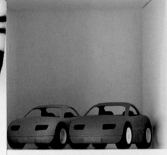
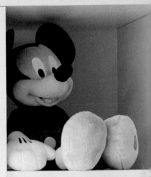
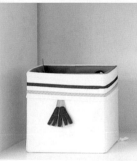
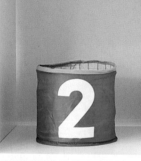
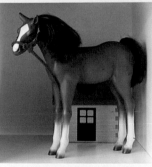
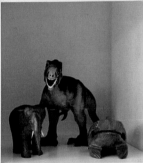
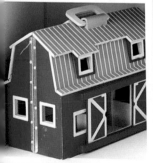
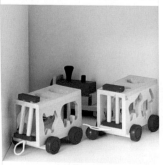
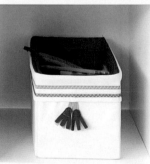
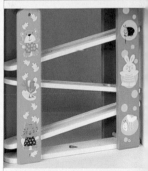
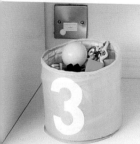
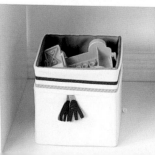
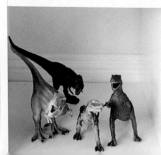
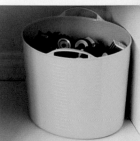

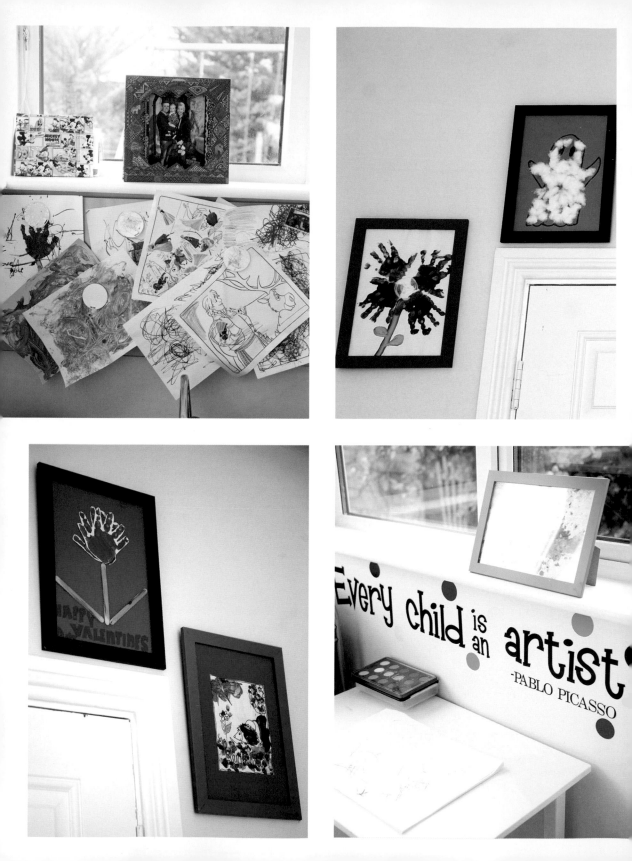

The art corner in our playroom is my favourite – we bought Ollie a little table and chair, again from IKEA, it was so affordable. Over his desk, I placed an art decal that says 'Every child is an artist' – I got it on etsy.com. Apart from loving the quote, it adds a bright pop of colour to this corner of the room. He loves sitting at his own table to draw – I have learnt, though, that markers aren't my friend with a cream carpet! Now we buy him those twistable crayons that look like markers. If we're painting, I just make sure he has his plastic apron on and I've newspaper down – that way he can mess away and enjoy it.

For storing his paints, paper and crayons, I got bright yellow boxes and labelled each one. I keep them on a little trolley beside his desk so that he can easily reach them.

You can add bold colour to the walls of a playroom by framing favourite paintings that your kids have created themselves. I have frames with clear plastic, rather than glass, and if your kids are old enough they can help mount their pieces. If a painting is too large for a frame, try cutting it up into sections, framing each one and then hanging the frames together on a wall to recreate it like a mosaic.

On another wall in the playroom, we have a magnetic board that Ollie can put his drawings on. If you run out of displaying space, get a big scrapbook and stick pictures into the book with a glue stick – you'll be glad you kept them in years to come when your babies aren't babies anymore!

 TIP *Before buying any furniture, go online to see if you can buy second hand – you can be so lucky and nab something that's exactly what you're looking for at half the price.*

BOOKS

We love books and I'm always encouraging Ollie to read. We used to have lots of books in different places – in drawers, on shelves, in buckets. So I knew I wanted to create something where Ollie could see and reach his books easily. I went on to Pinterest and searched for 'kids book units'. (By the way, Pinterest is amazing for getting all sorts of inspiration and ideas.)

I saw a photo of a bookcase that I loved and went in search of something similar. In the end, I got it made by an Irish company called Wooden Gifts Ireland. I just showed them the pic, they made it, delivered it to my house and assembled it, too. I also got a really cute 'Shhhh' sign made to go over it – you could get a sign saying whatever you liked. The bookshelf came in white, as I wanted. Afterwards, we decided to paint the sign blue, so I bought a little sample pot of paint, and that was all I needed to paint it twice. It's really neat and safely secured onto the wall. I'm thrilled with it, and it definitely encourages Ollie to reach for the books as they're facing out. It looks great in the room too.

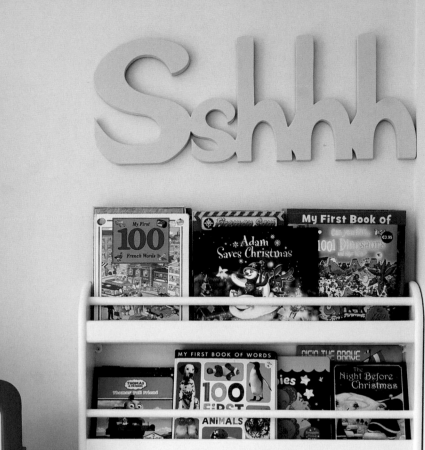

Sshhh

My First **100** French Words

Adam Saves Christmas

My First Book of

100l Dinosaurs

MY FIRST BOOK OF WORDS

THOMAS & FRIENDS
Thomas' Tall Friend

100 FiRST

ANiMALS

The **Night Before Christmas**

All the Ways I Love You

THE **GRUFFALO**

Baby Jesus

I'm Ready to Read with **Mickey**

Freddy Buttons and the **Apple Bandits**

THE **GRUFFALO** and other stories

MICKEY MOUSE A Magical Story

Fairy Welcome Guide

The Smartest **GIANT** in Town

my baby's journal

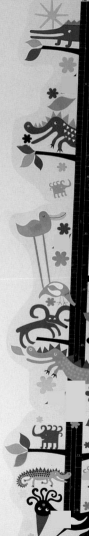

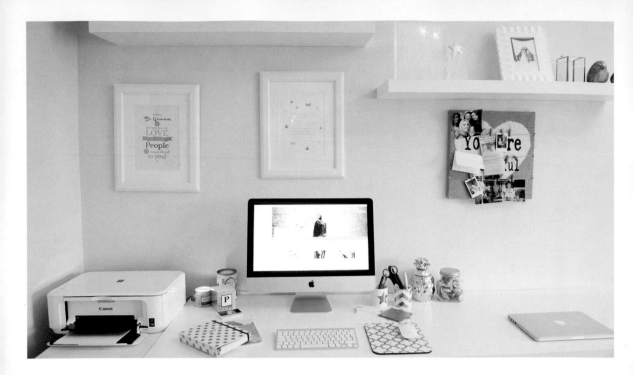

OFFICE

I'm gold obsessed. If it's brass and shiny, I want it. I love gold for interiors and knew this was something I wanted to focus on for my office.

I had lots of lovely prints with gold foil on them, so that started the idea of a featured gold wall in one area of the room. It's probably my favourite spot to relax, read, sit and think. I believe it's really important to have a space somewhere that's just for you, that you love.

I shopped around for gold frames, which I got mainly from TK Maxx. They have a great mixture of quirky interior stuff. I then got an old cream armchair, which worked perfectly in the corner, and threw a bright cushion on it to add some colour. I also found two really old side tables, which looked great too. I didn't even bother to paint them. I put some candles, a picture frame and always some flowers on the tables, and there you have it – a cosy sanctuary.

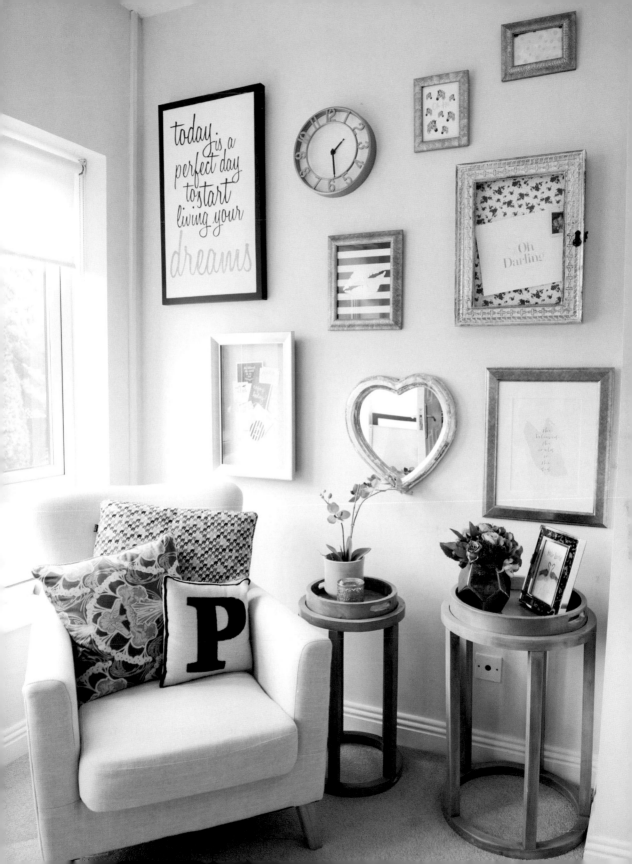

I believe it's really important to have a space somewhere that's just for you, that you love.

I kept the gold theme throughout my office with a large gold mirror and some gold accessories on my desk. I chose bright turquoise chairs and cushions that popped with shades of pink. I adore the colour combo of gold, pink and turquoise.

For storage, I have the same IKEA units that I got for Ollie's playroom except mine look a little different as I have doors on some of the cubbyholes to hide my paperwork, and I have some really handy pull-out canvas baskets in others to keep my bits and bobs in.

Above the unit, I decided to frame some of my favourite magazine covers that I've appeared on over the years – not because I love looking at myself, but because it's nice to remember all of those special moments in your life, how far you've come, and how hard you've worked. It's kind of like an athlete displaying their trophies, I suppose!

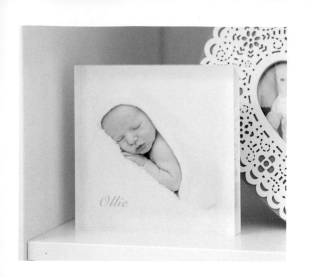

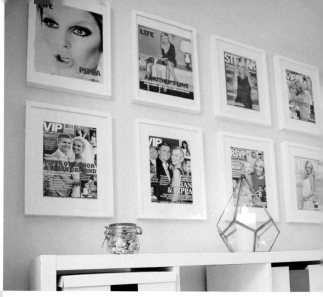

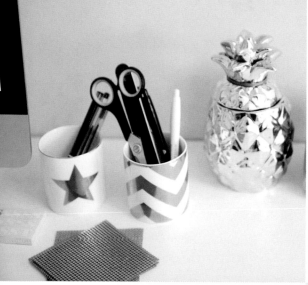

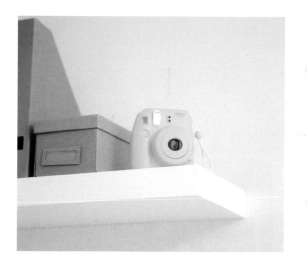

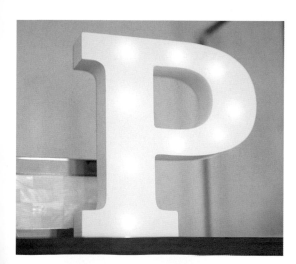

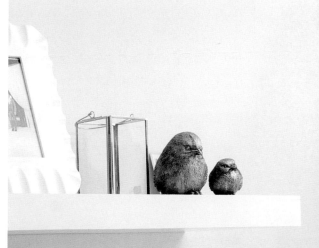

BEDROOM

Your bedroom is just as important as the living room – after all, it's where you spend most of your time. You should be able to shut the door at night and love the space you're in.

When it comes to the arrangement of items in a bedroom, balance and proportion is a really important factor. You need also to feel calm and relaxed in your bedroom so make sure your bed is as comfortable as possible. You should replace your mattress every eight years and if you can see a visible dip in the middle, it creaks or you can feel its springs, then it's definitely time to change your mattress. Choosing the right bedding is important too, and in my opinion, luxurious sheets, downy pillows and large cushions are not unnecessary expenditure, but an investment.

 TIP *Bed linen can be so expensive, especially in super king size, so get it in the sales. I find the January sales are best for picking up linen and towels at a fraction of the usual price.*

When it comes to colours, I like to go for crisp, white sheets with soft neutral-coloured blankets and bed covers, which you can easily add to or alter with a dash of colour from a cushion, or perhaps flowers on the bedside table.

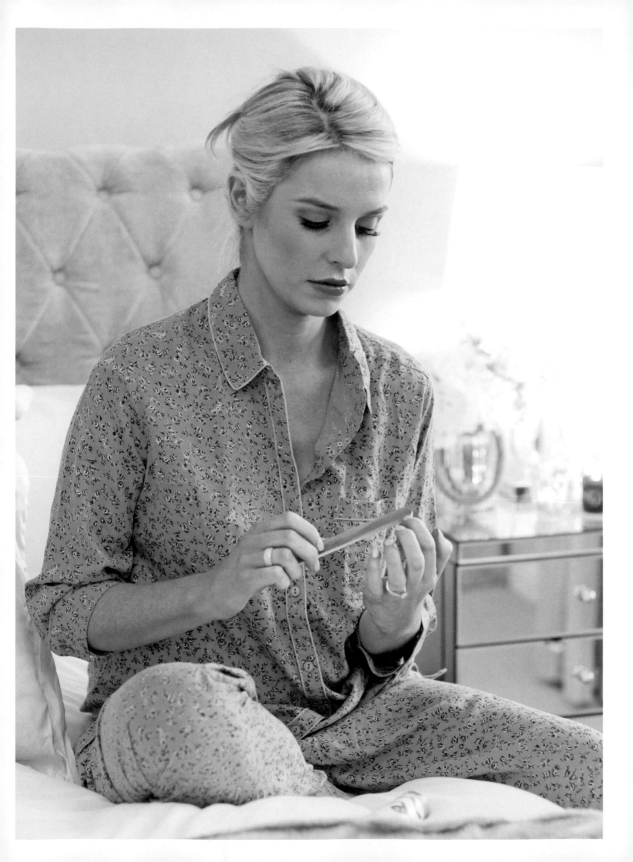

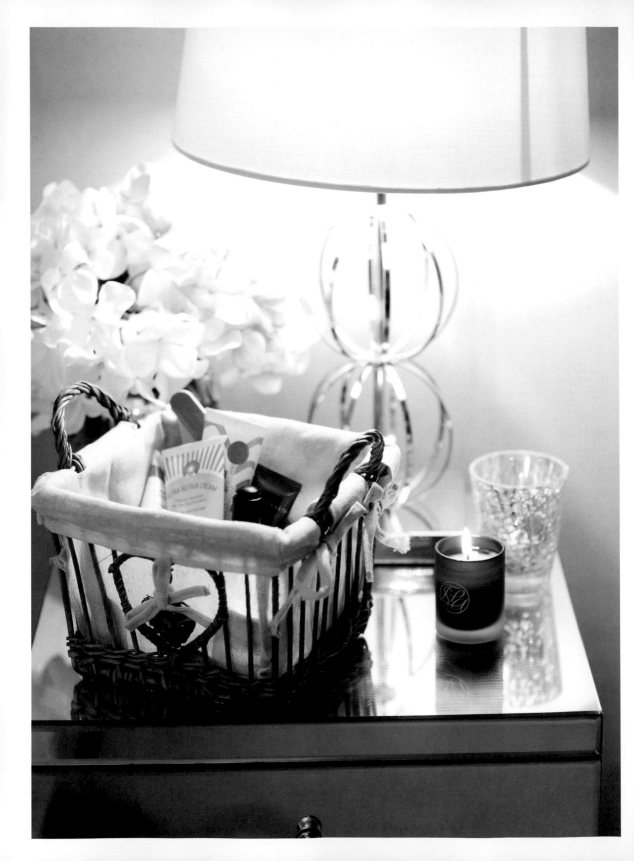

I like to have nightstands or side tables on either side of the bed. Here's what I keep on my nightstand:

- a low-lit lamp.

- a scented candle. I love the smell of lavender in a bedroom as it's so relaxing. Try burning some lavender oil or candles just before you get into bed to help soothe the mind.

- flowers, when possible. A little bunch of flowers in a bedroom is such a lovely touch. Not only do they smell beautiful, but when you wake up in the morning you'll instantly smile at the sight of them.

- I keep most of my nighttime skin products in a little wicker basket by my bed. This means it's less time standing in the bathroom when you're tired and just want to get into bed. You can do your moisturizing and creams in bed at your leisure, and I find the routine of putting on the various products before bed calming and a good end to the day. I have my eye cream, night cream, night oil, hand cream, nail file and lip balm all in the basket beside me. It looks very sweet too!

Mirrors, like elsewhere, create the feeling of space and help to reflect light. Lighting should be gentle and relaxing. Subtle light gives a romantic feeling to the room – I personally prefer low lighting from lamps rather than lights fixed into the ceiling.

I find the routine of putting on various products before bed calming and a good end to the day.

SWITCHING OFF

Speaking of soothing the mind, I think it's really important to have some rules for phones and laptops in bed. Life is so hectic, I know, and it can be so hard to switch off in the evening, especially from social media and emails. I now give myself a cut off point in the evenings where I no longer check my emails or look at social media. Your brain needs time to be calm, still and recharge for the next day. Otherwise it's like a vicious daily cycle, you're on overdrive, you're not getting enough sleep, then you're tired again the next day. And it really doesn't add to the romance to be constantly on your phone in bed!

We have a TV in our room and there's nothing nicer than cuddling up to watch a movie but again, try to limit the TV time in your bedroom too. Read a book, make a list of goals, meditate. Just relax and be still. Try it, you'll be amazed at how relaxed you'll feel after you get into the routine of taking time out!

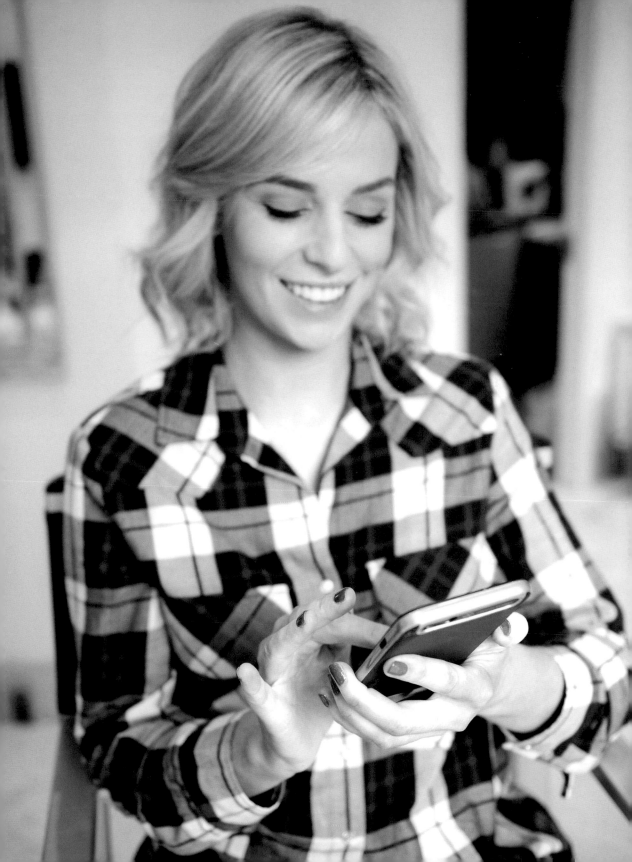

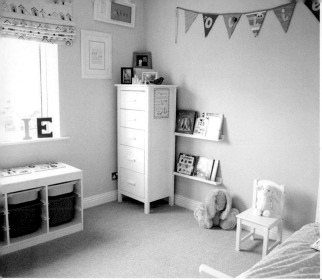
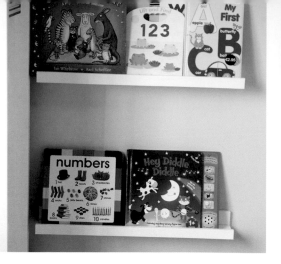
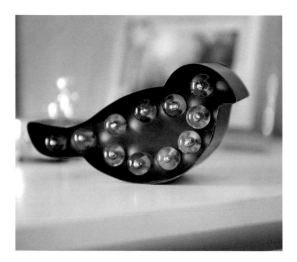
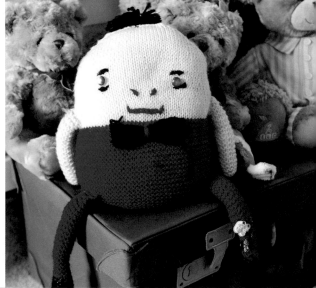
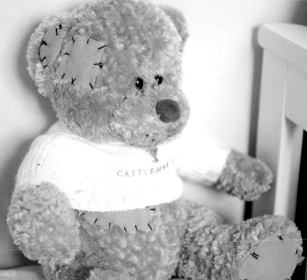
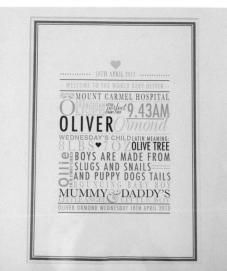

CHILD'S BEDROOM

Ollie loves his little bedroom. He had quite a neutral nursery in our last house, so now that this one is blue and colourful he loves spending time in there. I decided to paint the walls blue, although I was a little nervous about it at the beginning as I had tested one blue previously and I felt it darkened the room. I found this blue by Dulux called 'Cape Cod' which was the perfect shade for me. It's a fresh bright blue. That particular range of paint is designed for kids' rooms and they are really easy to wipe clean – just in case any budding artists have accidents. Thankfully, we've had no incidents of drawing on the walls – yet!

When Ollie was born, we invested in a cot bed that has served him brilliantly. We turned the cot into a bed just after his second birthday and he absolutely loved his 'big bed' from day one. It's low on the ground and not too big and scary. He'll probably get another year or so out of it before he's too tall, but I'd highly recommend buying a cot that turns into a bed, it's very convenient.

Ollie has some toys in his room that are kept in a low storage unit in red buckets that he can easily get to. It's been a good idea keeping a small selection of toys in his room as some mornings he'll wake up and happily play on his own before coming into us to give us our wake up call. That extra half hour makes all the difference!

He has a little book corner and chair in his room too. The ledges are actually picture frame ledges from IKEA – a brilliant (and cheap) alternative to buying a bookshelf. They're really neat and easy to attach to the wall. We hung them low so he can reach them whenever he wants.

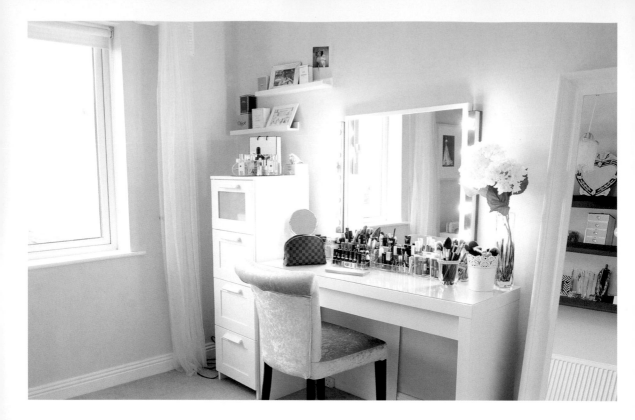

BEAUTY ROOM

My 'getting ready room', as I like to call it! I love my beauty room as it's full of all my favourite personal bits and pieces. It's where I sit every morning to paint my face. It's also where I listen to music and try on outfits. And I can relax here and plan my day ahead.

My little room was a spare room – or a dumping ground, I should say! So, I decided to clear it out and make use of the small space I had. I added a neat dressing table and chair and my hubby mounted my mirror and lights – luckily he's a real handyman around the house. I love the strip of lighting around my mirror – lots of lighting companies do them or, again, you can get very affordable ones from IKEA.

To store my make-up products, I have a tall chest of drawers in the room, too. The drawers are very deep, which is great for tall bottles so you can store them upright rather than flat and thrown in on top of one another. I try to keep some order to the drawers, so I'll keep hair products in one, skincare products in another, tans and mitts in another and so on.

On top of my dressing table, I keep things I use regularly like my make-up brushes, foundations and certain lipsticks. I keep my brushes in old candle jars or plant pots – they make brilliant holders. I put my make-up in plastic see-through cases – you can get these in nearly every homewear store now and mine are mainly from TK Maxx.

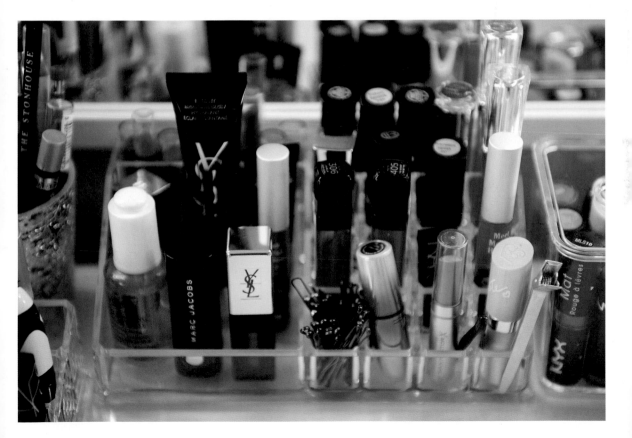

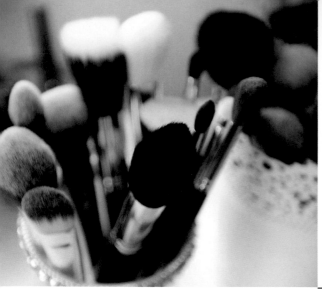

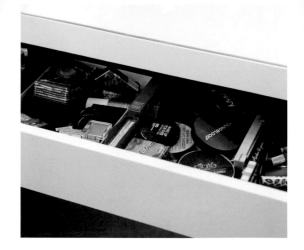

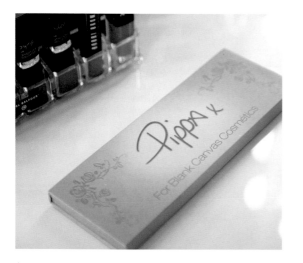

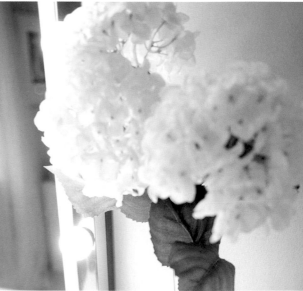

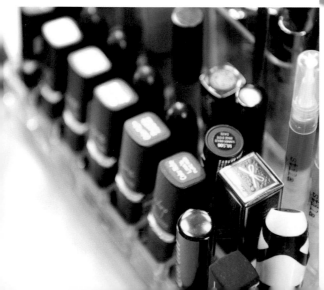

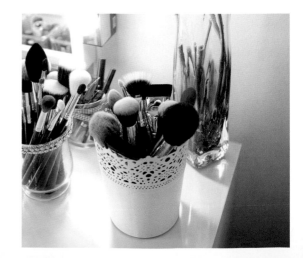

On my table, I have a tall thin vase (so as not to take up much room) with some artificial flowers. I prefer fresh flowers but artificial ones can look great too. If opting for artificial flowers try to get the more expensive silk ones. They just look much better and you'll have them for years in the long run.

My table has a pull out drawer, too, which is brilliant for extra storage. It's pretty shallow but can still fit a lot of smaller items. Originally, I had my make-up loosely inside but quickly it got very cluttered with everything mixed up resulting in me being able to find nothing. I decided to put in some dividers by using my old Glossyboxes – these are the perfect depth and work brilliantly for separating your make-up into different categories.

TIP *Did you know all of your make-up and skin products have a sell-by date? On the back you'll see a little symbol that looks like a container with either 6M, 12M or 24M on it. This is the product's best-by date. Use by 6, 12 or 24 months after opening. Beyond that date, your make-up or skincare lotion might not work as well or could even cause irritations or infections.*

Mascaras should definitely be changed every three months and don't share mascaras with friends, as the wand harbours a host of bacteria that can cause eye infections in others. So, try to remember when you open something, and stick to using it within the number of months recommended on the back.

PERFUME

I'm a perfume lover. I definitely have different scents I opt for, depending on the time of year. I have a couple that I always love and consistently go back to wearing.

- **Coco Mademoiselle** by Chanel – I love this all year round. It was my wedding day scent, too, so it holds special memories. I love wearing it with the matching body lotion and hairspray.

- **Pomegranate Noir** by Jo Malone – I usually buy a small bottle of this each winter. It's very distinctive and reminds me of Christmas.

- **Velvet Orchid** by Tom Ford – Tom Ford fragrances are among my favourites for both men and women. Velvet Orchid is quite strong and powerful, so it's a scent I usually keep for evenings.

- **Chance Eau Fraîche** by Chanel – this is my summer scent, it's really fruity and fresh.

The scent of a perfume changes continually when you're wearing it, so what you love at first might not be your thing an hour or so later. When trying perfumes, it's a good idea to wait an hour or two before you buy one. As well as changing over time, a scent can differ from person to person as it reacts with our own natural oils to produce a unique scent.

If ever you find a really nice scent but it always seems to fade it might be because you bought the eau de toilette. It's a lot cheaper, but it won't last as long as the eau de parfum. All fragrances have different levels of scented oils and the higher the concentration of those oils the longer a scent lasts on the skin.

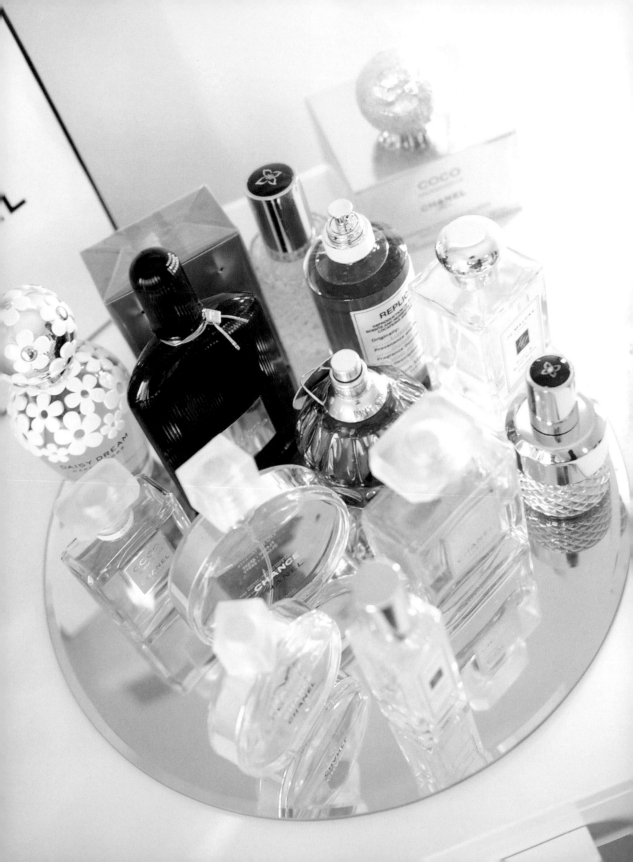

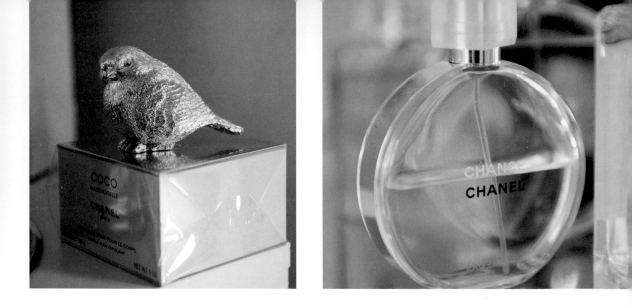

Eau de toilette

With a lighter concentration of scented oils, eau de toilette lasts for around two or three hours max. It's great if you like to change your perfume a few times during the day.

Eau de parfum

Eau de parfum has a higher concentration of aromatic oils, so it lasts much longer. It is more expensive, but you'll use less and it'll last for several hours.

Parfum

The most expensive of them all, parfum, or pure perfume, has around a 20 to 40 per cent concentration of scented ingredients, so it should last you all day. Don't overdo it though – it's the strongest stuff, so you only need a couple of drops.

I like to maximize my perfume by layering it. Use a scented shower gel and body lotion first thing in the morning, and apply a few drops of parfum before you dash out of the door. Keep the eau de toilette version in your bag so you can refresh the fragrance regularly throughout

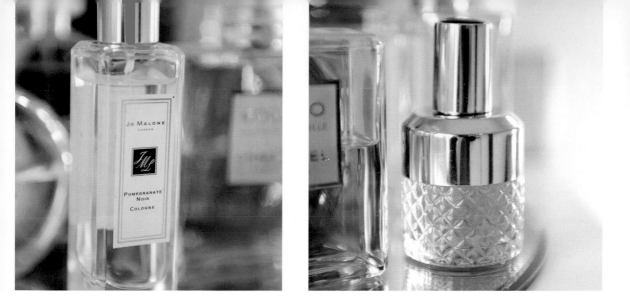

the day. And where should you spritz yourself? Pulse points – so, on your wrists, inside your elbows, the nape of your neck, even in the crease behind your knees.

There's so many to choose from it can be quite overwhelming, I know, but fragrances are often divided into four categories: floral (think fresh-cut flowers), fresh (to include citrus and fruit), oriental (to include sweet spices and vanilla) and woody (such as sandalwood and amber). If you're not sure what's what, ask for assistance at the perfume counter. Make a note of which types of smells you like – it could be cinnamon, apple, blossom or even autumnal leaves – this will all help to work out which fragrances are right for you.

Make sure you don't try too many at once, though. Most people can only cope with three or four before they become 'fragrance blind'. If you overdo it, grab a fresh coffee – the smell of coffee beans helps clear your nose.

And once you've bought your perfume, how should you store it? Upright and in its original box and somewhere fairly cool (not near a radiator). Exposure to light over a period of time will most definitely cause your fragrances to deteriorate.

SHOE STORAGE

Okay, I've mentioned my shoe wall already (more than once!) so, as you can tell, I'm pretty pleased with this latest addition to my getting ready room and very proud of my hubby for making it. Before we had this, most of my shoes covered the floor of the room that we needed to turn into a nursery for our impending arrival. It was so bad that I could hardly open the door!

So, with no more wardrobe space available, I asked my hubby if he could make shelves from the floor to the ceiling on one wall. Luckily for me, he obliged once again, and actually did it the very next day. I must be a pain to live with!

I chose plain white floating shelves – I didn't want ones with brackets showing. They'll need dusting regularly but I can cope with that! At least they look neat and tidy now.

It's such a simple but effective idea if you're stuck for shoe storage like me. I keep most of my heels and trainers on display. My long boots are kept in boxes in the wardrobe along with any expensive shoes, which I keep stuffed with tissue in their boxes. Not that I've many designer shoes; I've a few, but I'm a high street gal all the way.

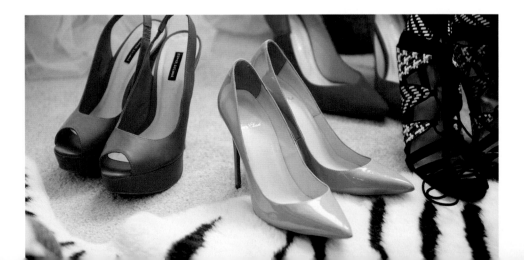

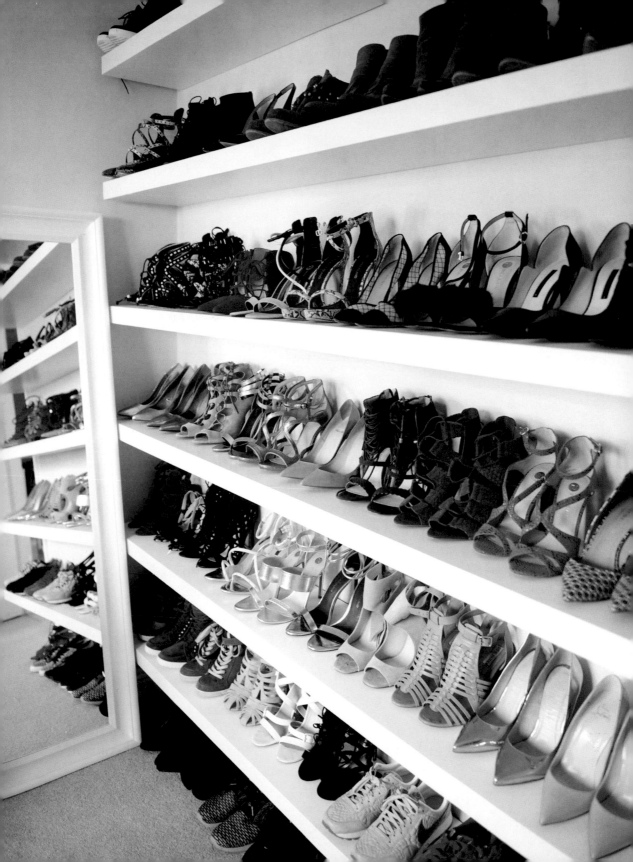

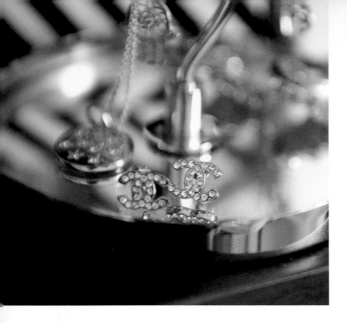
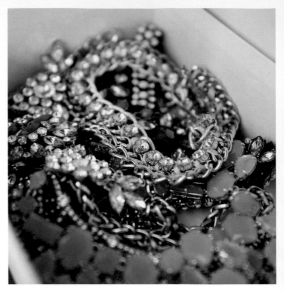

JEWELLERY

From statement necklaces and cocktail rings to dainty chains and earrings, I love collecting jewellery. I store it mainly on two shelves in my beauty room. I like buying quirky little jewellery boxes and holders simply because they look cute on display, but if you've no system to storing your jewellery it can easily turn into a tangled mess. There's nothing more annoying than wanting to wear a certain chain with an outfit but you just can't find it! Time to organize your jewellery.

First, go through every single piece you have and categorize each one. Then start organizing!

Bin/charity pile

If a costume ring is tarnished, throw it out.

Give away

If you feel you've grown out of something and you know you'll never wear it again, don't hang on to it, give it to someone who will enjoy it.

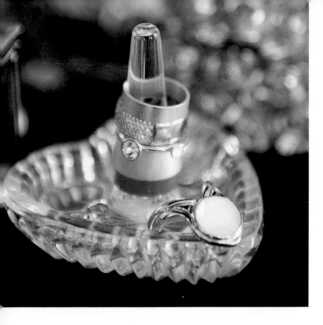

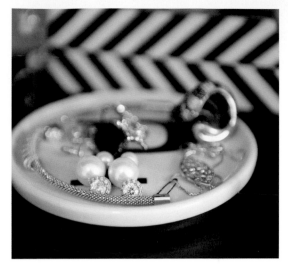

Statement necklaces

These aren't something I wear every day, so I keep them together, flat and neatly packed in a see-through box.

Dainty everyday chains

For these, I bought a little jewellery tree from Marks and Spencer. It's perfect for hanging your delicate pieces and it means you can see them easily every morning.

Rings

For my wedding and eternity rings, I have one special crystal ring holder, which my mum gave me, that I keep these on at nighttime. It's good to have one dedicated spot for holding your expensive or special items. I keep my other rings all together in a little box.

Small stud earrings

I keep these together on a little plate, which makes it really easy to see and reach for them.

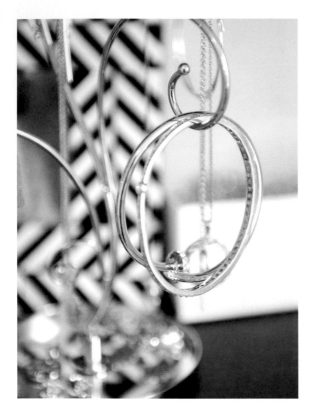
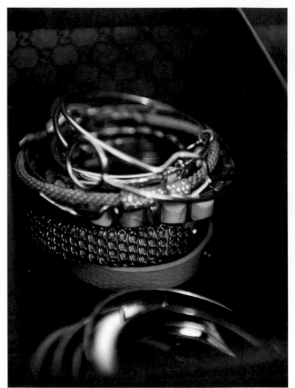

Extras

I like to keep my other earrings and bracelets in a jewellery pouch behind my door. It's a big holder with lots of different plastic compartments. I bought this in Primark years ago and it's been such a nifty storage piece. I hung a hook on the back of my door to hold it.

 TIP *If you're stuck for hanging space for either jewellery, belts or scarves, look behind doors and inside wardrobes to see where you could hang extra hooks. For things that don't weigh much try the sticky adhesive hooks for convenience.*

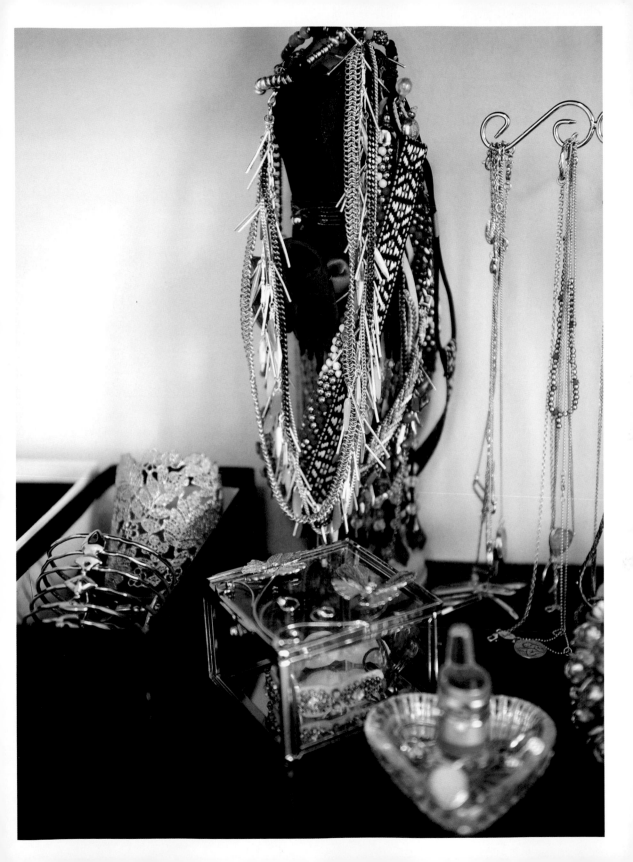

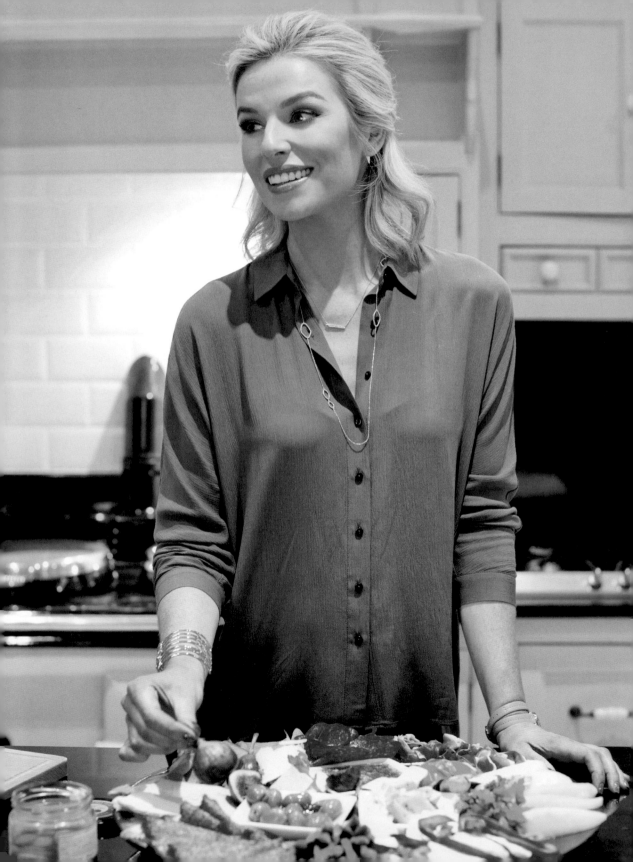

CHAPTER EIGHT

SIMPLE ENTERTAINING

It's great to have family and friends over. Whether it's a special occasion or just a get-together with people you like to spend time with, I love the intimacy of meeting up at home. I feel you get to chat and interact with your guests more when you're at your own place.

You might love the idea of having friends over but feel a bit daunted when it comes to preparing food or cooking. I'm definitely not the best chef in the world – I love nothing more than being served in a restaurant – but when it comes to cooking for guests, I have a few foolproof tips and tricks that have helped me over the years.

Before rushing off and buying food for the occasion, think carefully about the kind of food you want to serve. Is it a special occasion or just a casual dinner party? Are you going for a formal dinner, relaxed, home-cooked food with friends and family, or a drinks party with nibbles? How many people are you inviting? If it's more than six or eight, are you comfortable with cooking dinner for that number? More to the point, have you room at your table to seat everyone? If the answer is no, then consider doing finger food or maybe tapas (I'll show you how to do that shortly).

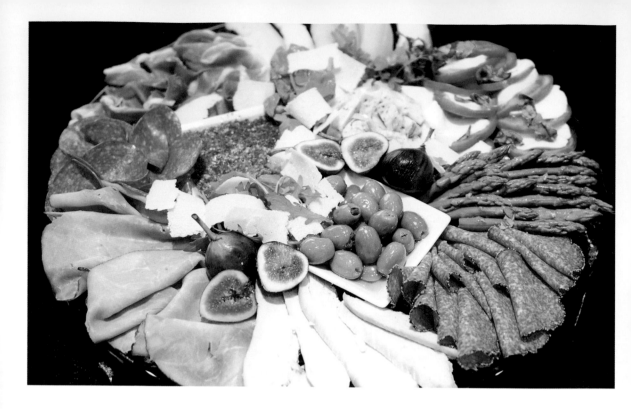

You might want to go all-out with a cheffy menu, but be realistic about what you can make at home, especially if you want to chat to your guests when they arrive. You don't want to be stuck in the kitchen in a mad flap when you could be enjoying yourself! Think practically: it might be difficult to cook ten lamb shanks at once in a regular-sized oven, for example, so don't even try. I always go for a menu that isn't too complicated, that can be prepared in advance and doesn't require multiple cooking pots. For me, entertaining should be simple and relaxed.

PARTY PLATTER

If I have a large crowd coming round for a drinks party, my party piece is a large hors d'oeuvre platter of finger food. Not only does this look impressive but it's so simple to prepare and can be done in advance. I have a nice large platter but you could also use a large bread board or

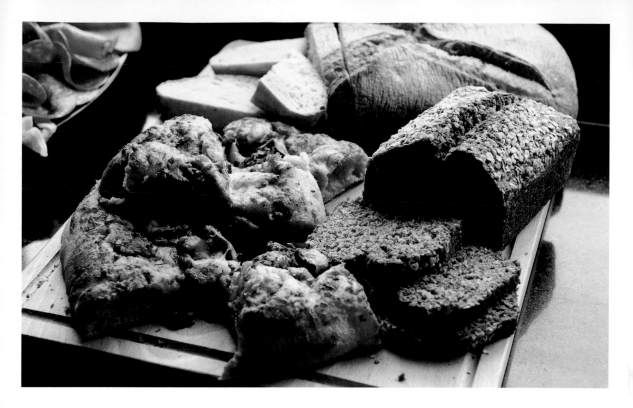

two. For my platter, I buy cold meats (such as salami and parma ham), cheeses (I like shavings of parmesan and slices of mozarella), fruits (like melon and figs), veggies (I love asparagus and artichoke hearts), rocket leaves, herbs and a few stuffed olives.

I'll put pesto and chutney into little bowls, and arrange everything so that foods that complement each other are next to each other. Mozzarella and tomatoes are a classic combination and the halved figs add a splash of colour. I serve some fresh bread on the side that has been warmed in the oven.

I love this dish (and so do my guests!) – it looks so colourful and is much healthier than crisps and peanuts. Saying that, do make sure you know your guests' dietary requirements in advance as you could easily make this a vegetarian-only platter or replace the meat with fish or shellfish.

Oven-poached lemon tarragon chicken

Serves 6–8

Chicken makes a great dish as most people like it, it's readily available, not too expensive, low in calories and children love it too. I prefer to buy free range, fresh chicken.

This is a simple recipe that my aunt Freda gave to me – she's another amazing chef in my family! This is a delicate-tasting dish that will suit all ages and tastes for a lovely family dinner. It's really clever because you can use the same technique for three different meals, depending on the occasion.

For the chicken

- 6–8 boneless chicken breasts
- 2 sticks of celery, each cut into 3
- 1 large carrot, cut into 4
- 1 small onion, quartered
- 3 sprigs of tarragon, plus a sprig for garnishing
- 2 sprigs of parsley
- 2 bay leaves
- A few black peppercorns
- Juice of 1 lemon, plus a slice of lemon rind for garnishing
- 1 chicken stock cube dissolved in 500 ml boiling water
- 300 ml white wine
- Cornflour

TIP *if you don't have every ingredient on the list, don't worry.*
If you don't have fresh tarragon, a little dried will do but only a
little, as dried herbs are stronger than fresh. You can also substitute
water for the wine.

1 Preheat your oven to 350°F/180°C. Put the chicken breasts in a ovenproof casserole dish or roasting pan making sure that they are not sitting on top of each other or they won't cook properly. Then add the vegetables, herbs, peppercorns, lemon juice and slice evenly around.

2 Dissolve the stock cube in 500 ml boiling water and add the white wine. Pour over the chicken breasts and vegetables making sure that they are covered with the liquid – you may need to add a little hot water depending on the size of your dish.

3 Cover the dish with tinfoil and poach for 30–35 minutes in the oven, making sure the chicken is cooked right through and there is no sign of any pink.

4 When the chicken is cooked, take it out of the oven, and let it rest in the liquid for a few minutes. Strain the stock into a pan, discarding the vegetables. Bring the stock to boil and reduce it by about half to give it a stronger flavour. To thicken it slightly add a little cornflour (about a tablespoon). I blend the cornflour with a little cold water first and then stir it into the liquid, letting it simmer for three minutes to cook through.

5 I like to serve one chicken breast per person, then spoon over a little thickened jus, with the remaining jus in a jug on the side. Garnish with the slice of lemon rind and tarragon. Serve with new potatoes and vegetables. It looks, smells and tastes delicious!

See the next page for another two ideas based on this poached chicken method.

Creamy tarragon and lemon chicken with rice

Serves 6–8

Additional ingredients for sauce

- Juice of half a lemon (optional)
- 300 ml single cream
- 1 tbsp fresh chopped or ½ tbsp dried tarragon
- Salt and white pepper

1 Prepare the chicken exactly as the previous recipe (steps 1–3). When the chicken is cooked all the way through leave it to cool in the liquid until manageable, then remove the breasts and chop into cubes.

2 Strain the liquid into a large saucepan, discarding the vegetables. If you like a really lemony flavour, add the juice of half a lemon. Simmer until you reduce the liquid by half. Add the single cream and thicken with a little cornflour (about a tablespoon), simmering for three minutes until it is cooked through.

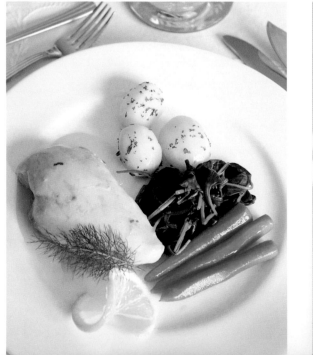
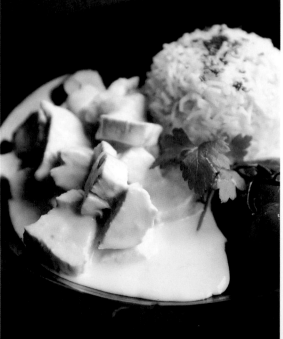

3 Season to taste with a pinch of salt and white pepper and a tablespoon of fresh chopped tarragon or half a tablespoon of dried tarragon. Then add in the chicken and heat through. Serve with boiled rice and a green salad.

Just having a girly daytime lunch?

Serve your creamy tarragon chicken mix on a large lettuce leaf, maybe with some cold pasta or cous cous. Take a couple of dessert spoonfuls of the cold, reduced chicken stock and mix it with some shop-bought mayonnaise, with a little grated lemon rind and some freshly chopped tarragon. Flavouring the mayonnaise depends on your own personal preference; the poached chicken will already taste great. This is so delicious and a perfect girly lunch favourite of mine.

For dessert I suggest something really simple again – a beautifully displayed cheese board or fresh fruit salad and cream. No need for fuss and you can have it done way in advance. Just cover with cling film until you're ready.

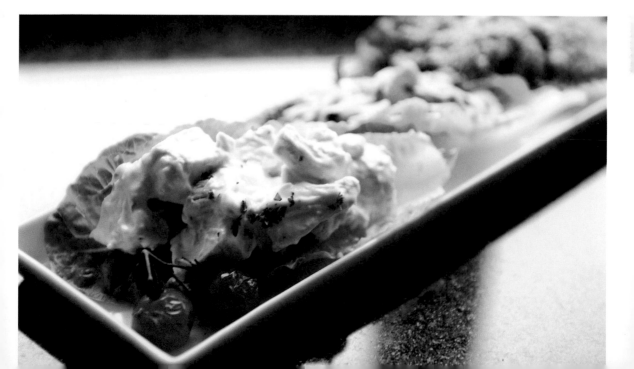

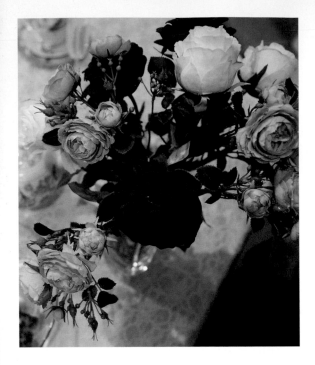
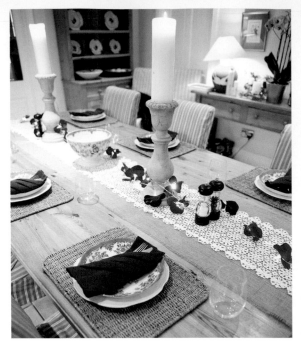

DRESSING THE TABLE

- For a more formal dinner party, I love using my white table cloth and white napkins.

- A simple white flower display and small tea lights for candles can look so pretty and elegant. I like my table settings to be a bit like my style – simple!

- For a casual dinner get-together there's no need for the fancy table cloth. A table runner can be just as impressive and less formal. Chunky pillar candles will give your table a relaxed feel.

- Get a strip of battery-operated artificial flower lights to add a cosy girly touch.

- **TIP** *Go to a fabric shop and buy a strip of lace or whatever material you like – this is cheaper than buying a 'runner' from a department store, plus you'll have more choice if you make up your own.*

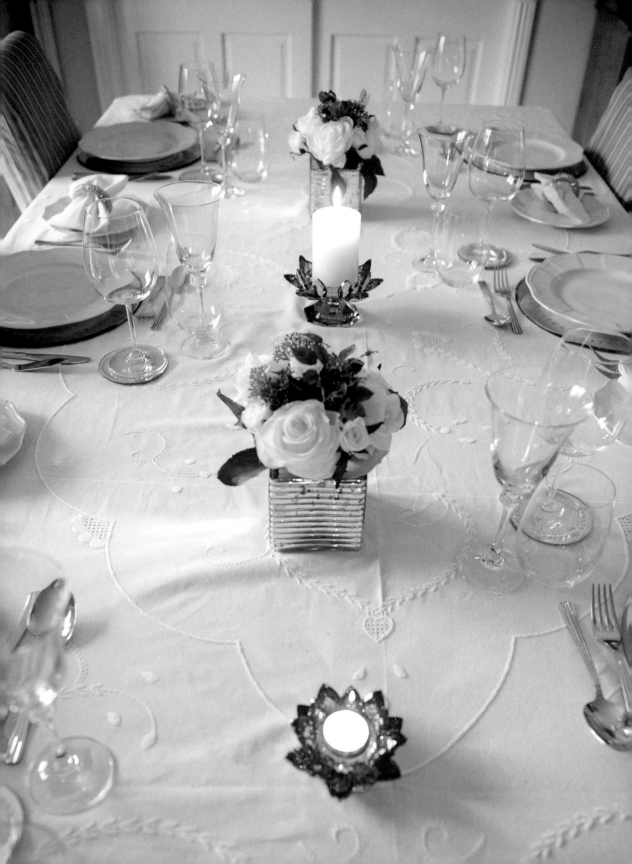

TOP HOSTING TIPS

Prepare as much as you can before your guests arrive so you too can enjoy the occasion. Here are some more tips on how to create the perfect party atmosphere with the minimum of stress:

- Choose an album or create a playlist of songs to set the mood. Put this on before the guests arrive as it helps the host to de-stress and creates a party atmosphere for the guests arriving.

- Don't leave getting ready yourself until the last minute. Do your make-up base earlier in the day. If blow-drying your hair, do it early and leave to set in velcro rollers.

- Saying that, wear your comfy clothes until an hour before your guests arrive. Don't attempt to cook or do any last-minute cleaning in your nice outfit.

- Light some scented candles half an hour before your guests arrive.

- Set up a little drinks area and have all of your glasses out, cleaned, polished and ready to go. Have ice in a bucket ready and lemons and limes pre-sliced.

- If you're serving nibbles like nuts or crisps before your dinner party, don't overdo it. You don't want your guests to be full on savoury snacks.

- Don't be in a rush to clear and clean plates the moment you've finished dinner. Hide them somewhere until your guests are gone!

- And remember, just relax and enjoy yourself! There's nothing more off-putting than an anxious or nervous host. Nobody expects perfection – this is meant to be fun!

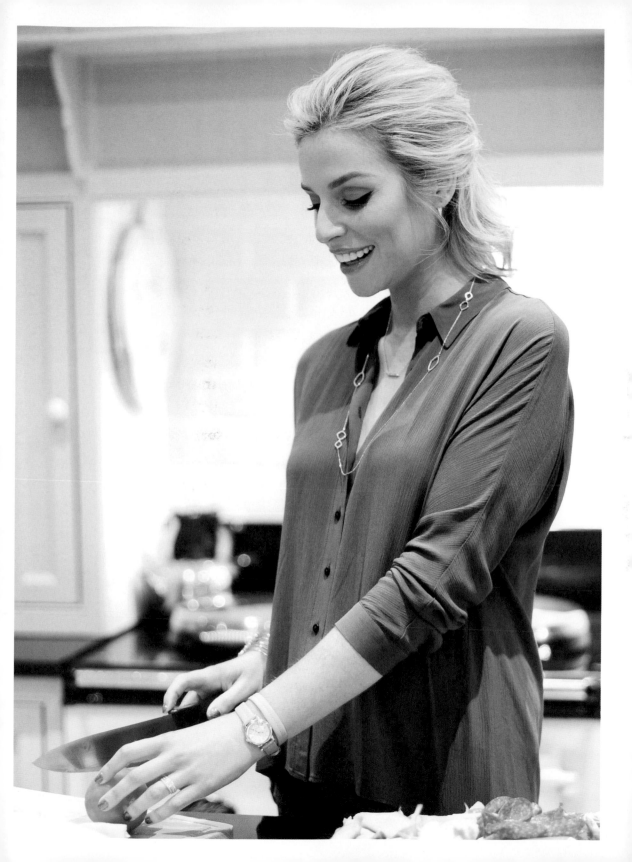

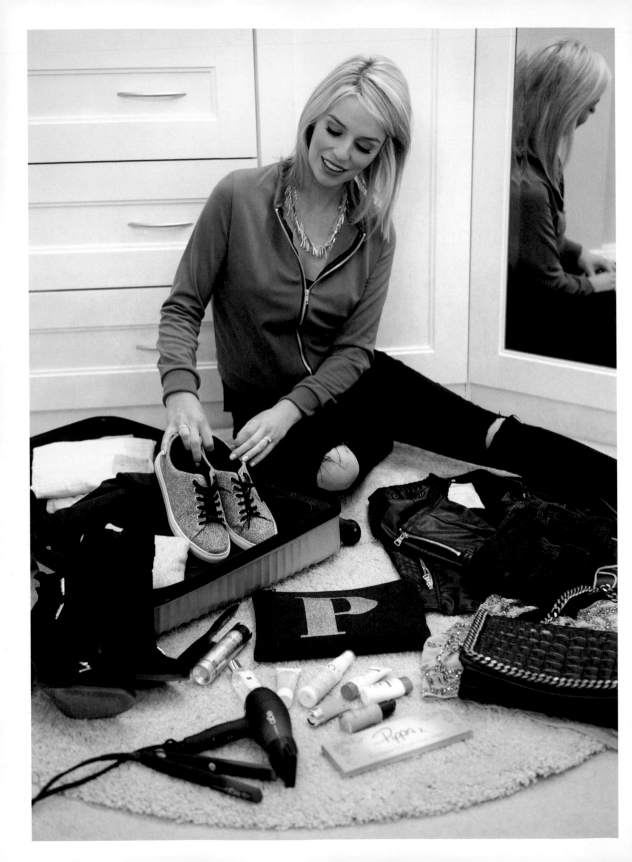

CHAPTER NINE

TRAVEL IN STYLE

I love to travel, whether it's a weekend away with the girls, a working trip, or a family holiday somewhere relaxing. Arriving is the fun bit but packing can be a bit of headache, as can the journey there and back, especially if you have little ones in tow!

I've done quite bit of travelling in my time, so when it comes to packing my stuff, I've pretty much got it sorted now. I always go for clothes and colours that I can mix and match, as well as the odd accessory, like a statement necklace or scarf, that can glam up an outfit and be squeezed into any bag.

Features on travelling with young children have always proved really popular on my blog so I've included some tips here. Preparation is key, as is making sure your little ones have lots to do if it's a really long journey. If you're off on holiday, though, try not to stress too much and just enjoy watching the world go by.

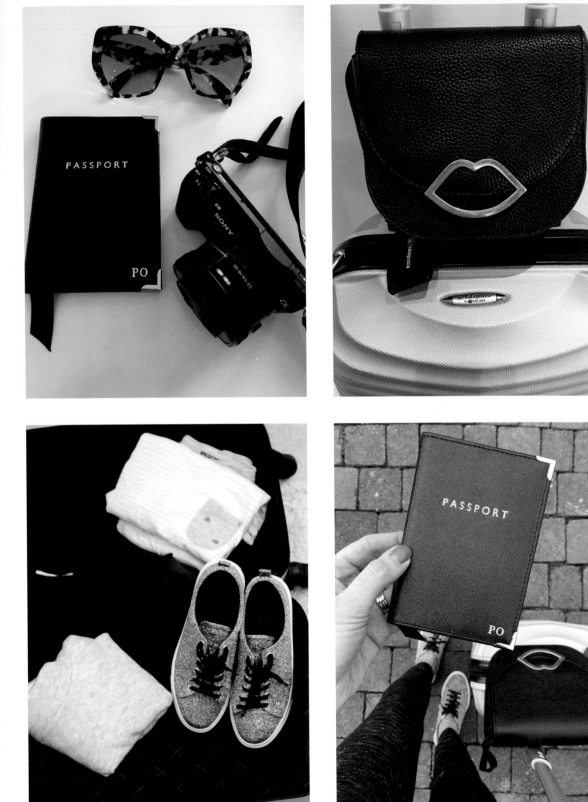

PACKING FOR A WEEKEND AWAY

We're all guilty of over-packing. It can be even trickier to pack when you're going away for just a weekend, but with a little forward planning I'll help you to pack like a pro! Here are a few suggestions:

Where are you going?

Think about where you're going and what you're doing. It sounds silly, but you'd be amazed how often people forget about it. They go into their routine and ignore the details. You might want to wear something light and comfortable for sight-seeing or mooching about in the day, for example. Remember to check the forecast because there's nothing worse than being caught out by a bit of rain! For a night out or a special occasion, you'll want to glam up so you could either mix or match what you have or bring a separate outfit.

Pick a colour scheme

Choose a couple of colours (say, grey and black) and then work everything around this. Lay your selection out on the bed, choose some accessories, and then try it all on. Don't just leave things to chance – make sure you're happy with your outfits from head to toe.

Reuse and renew

To minimize the amount you're packing, think about re-using some of the items you bring, such as shoes, jewellery and hats. For example, if you're travelling in a denim shirt and leather jacket, you could wear the same jacket at night with a cute, sparkly top.

Roll with it

Try rolling instead of folding your clothes – this takes less room and they're actually less likely to crease.

Size is everything

Take a medium-sized handbag that you can use day or night to save you bringing two. For toiletries, always have some minis on hand to pop in your bag for travelling. If you're flying and taking only hand luggage put your minis in a clear bag before you get to airport security. I have a mini hair dryer and mini straighteners that are so handy for packing as they're tiny but they're actually much better than the usual hotel hair dryer.

✳ **TIP** *If you don't want to iron something, use your hair dryer as an iron. This works a treat. Do it while you're wearing the item, just don't burn yourself! Or try hanging your clothes up in the bathroom while you're having a shower – the moisture in the air helps to uncrease the clothes.*

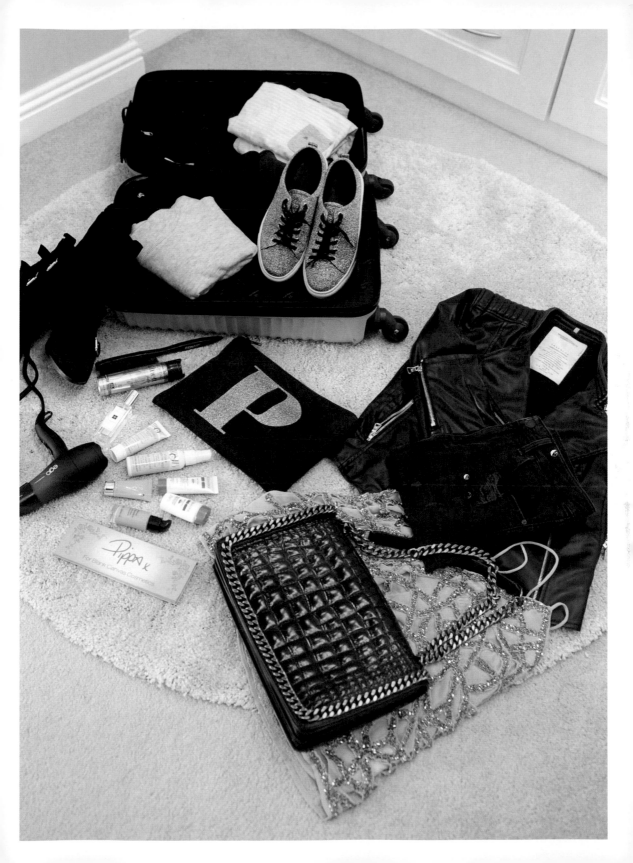

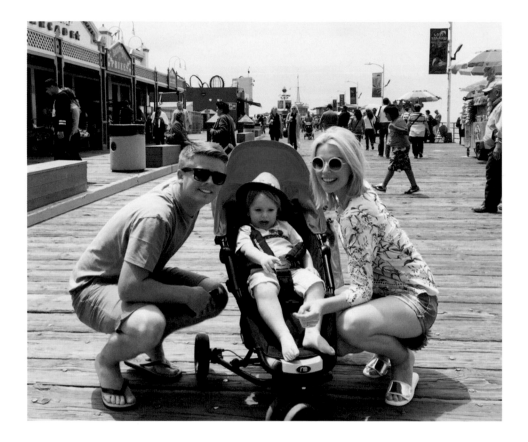

TRAVELLING WITH KIDS

When Ollie was nine months old we went on our first family holiday abroad … Boy, was there A LOT to think about beforehand. I made list after list. I'd never travelled with a baby before so I was extremely anxious and a little flustered about what to bring and what to expect.

Travelling with a baby is an exciting time but can also be terrifying for some parents as it can make travelling seem that little bit more complicated. Like anything, if you prepare properly, everything will run smoothly.

If it's your first time travelling with your baby, they will need their own passport. Follow the rules about the photograph to the absolute letter. You'll get through quite a few coins in the photo booth before you get a photo that ticks all the boxes, but if it's not absolutely perfect, it will be rejected by the authorities. A better alternative to a photo booth is having your baby's picture taken at a high-street photo development shop. They'll use a digital camera and will keep going until they get a suitable shot.

Don't do what I did and leave getting your baby's passport until the last minute. Give yourself plenty of time and room for error. You'll have enough to think about in the run-up to your trip.

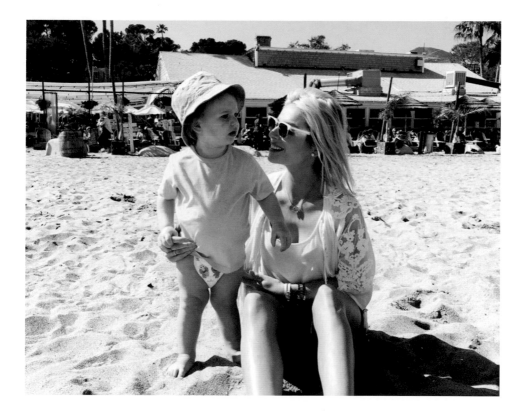

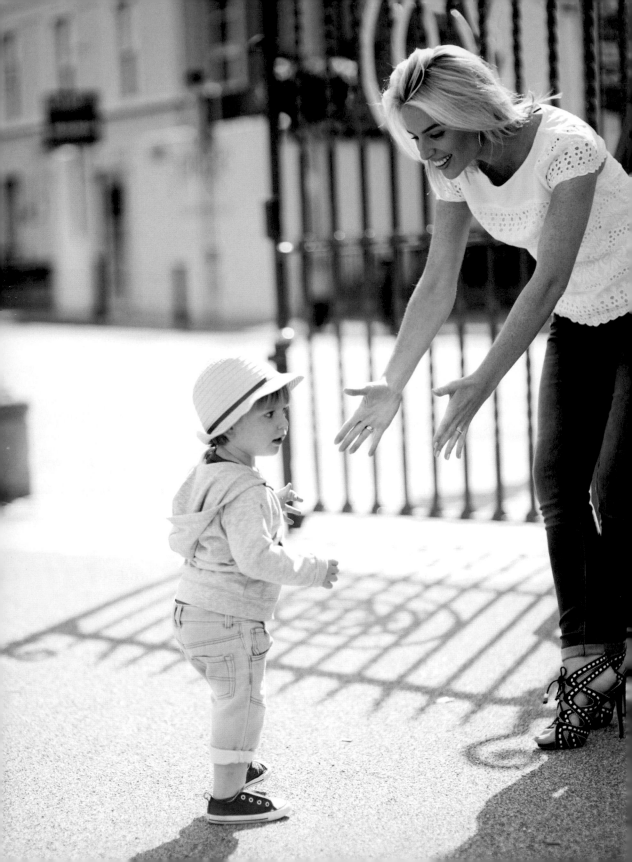

PACKING FOR KIDS

At some point nearly all parents wonder why their tiny baby needs more luggage than the average WAG. But most of us pack too much. Of course you need the essentials – nappies, wipes, formula milk and bottles if you're not breastfeeding, plus clothes. But unless you are heading for Outer Mongolia, you will find shops selling all these things.

We went to America on our first holiday, so I really didn't need to bring lots of extra things like rice cakes, yoghurts, etc. I could have lightened the load by just bringing the essentials for the flight, plus one day, just until I got to a shop. If only a specific brand will do for your baby, however, you might want to check that it's sold in the country you're going to and at what price.

Also check ahead to see if your accommodation has a washing machine, to cut down on clothes. Many hotels and resorts now offer bottle warmers and sterilizers. If not, sterilizing fluid or tablets are easier to pack than your giant steam sterilizer. I used Dr Brown sterilizing bags from Mothercare and I found them excellent. Very easy to use.

When it came to cots, we were staying in two different hotels that I knew had cots, but then we stayed with my brother for a while too. There was no cot there so we just bought one when we arrived. I had looked ahead and saw one on the Toys R Us site that was perfect and it was only €50 so I reckoned that it was worth doing this rather than bringing one over. It's also worth asking around to see if you can borrow one.

TIP *For toddlers, wrap up small toys for them to open on the journey – you'll be amazed at how excited and amused they'll be.*

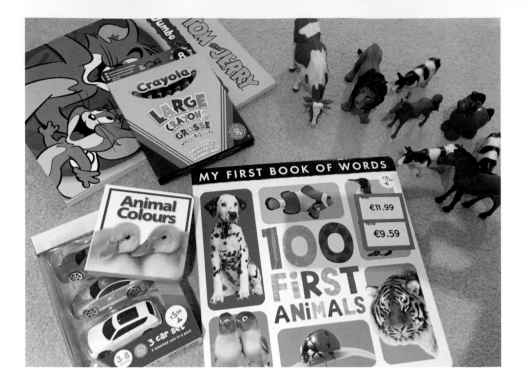

I absolutely adore the buggy I use at home but it comes in two parts and is too heavy to travel with. So I invested in a light foldable stroller, one that I could put up and down with one hand. It had a great lie back facility which meant Ollie could nap easily while out and about.

I also bought a travel bag for the buggy, again in Mothercare, which was invaluable when we were getting on and off planes and travelling. When it comes to toys, try to keep it to a minimum and be clever about what they'll actually use and like. I'll bring a couple of new toys, which makes for a nice surprise when I show them for the first time on the plane, along with his old favourites, like the bear he always sleeps with, a few fabric books and stacking beakers, etc.

Long-haul flights can be pretty harrowing with babies and small children – do try to book nighttime flights but don't worry too much about jet lag. Small babies' rhythms are much more adaptable than adults'.

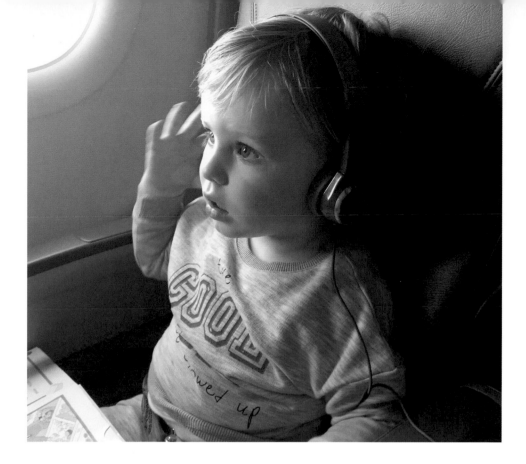

What else you'll need

- A change of clothes. Something comfortable like tracksuit bottoms with an elasticated waist band.

- Favourite blanket.

- Tablet or iPad. Pre-load with a movie and lots of new apps.

- Snacks, snacks and more snacks!

- Rice cakes, Liga, raisins, yoghurt in a pouch – easier than bringing a spoon for a pot – and some grapes.

- If you're worried about ears popping give them some milk when you're taking off or, if they're old enough, give them a lollipop to suck on. Both will help prevent their ears from popping.

HOW TO TRAVEL IN STYLE

Just because your travelling schedule may include trains, planes and automobiles, that doesn't mean your style should suffer. For me, comfort is key while travelling, but it's still possible to be comfortable without looking like you're in your Sunday loungewear.

I have a few friends that have been flight attendants and they always say if you want the chance to be upgraded on a flight always look smart. Good tip, I reckon! This doesn't mean you should wear leather trousers and high heels – there's a happy medium.

If flying long-haul, or if you're going on any long journey, I'd stay away from tight jeans. They'll restrict you, especially if you're trying to sleep comfortably. I'd opt for something like a pair of cuffed leg loose pants, preferably in a dark colour.

On top, I'd keep it casual but chic with a nice t-shirt and oversized knitted cardi – this will keep you warm on board too. Wear a bright scarf to add a pop of colour. It's a good idea to have a couple of layers.

For footwear, you want something easy to take off, especially for going through airport security – stay away from anything with tight laces or buckles. I usually wear my sparkly Sandro trainers travelling – yes, they're trainers, but they're what I call my snazzy trainers – and don't forget the little footsie socks to wear with them.

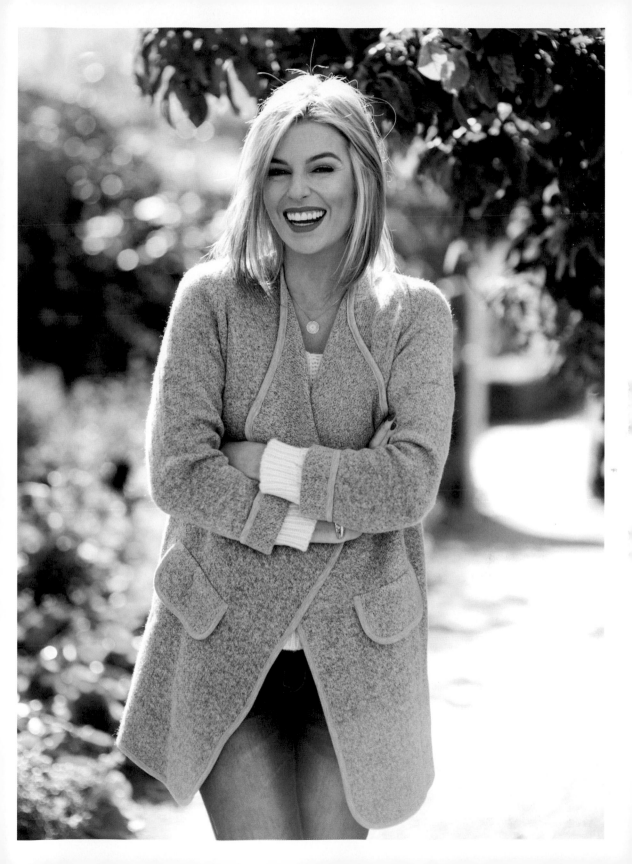

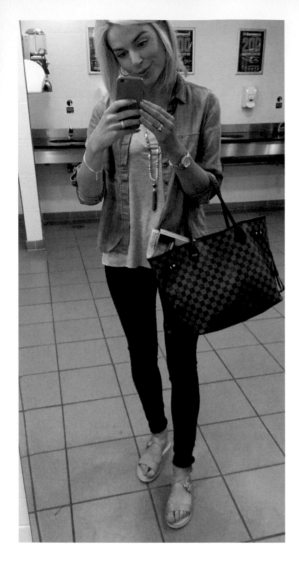

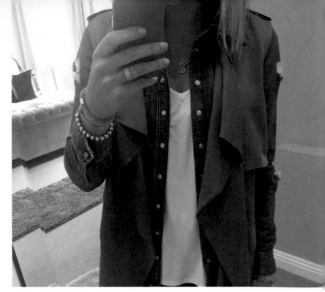

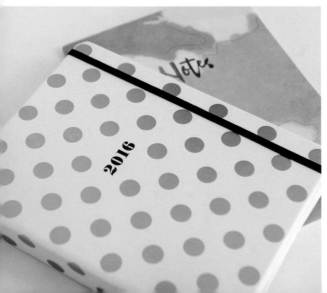

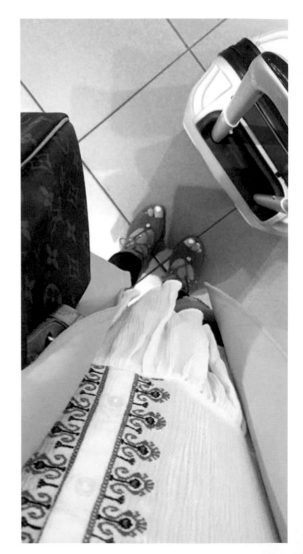

Keep your jewellery to a minimum – again it's only hassle going through airport security having to take bangles off, etc. Plus, if you're like me, your hands and fingers will swell while travelling so it's best just to wear the minimum. For a handbag, I usually bring a saddle-type bag that I can wear over my shoulder or across my body (especially handy if you're travelling with children as your hands will be free). A bag like this with one or two compartments is ideal as you can keep your passport and itinerary easily at hand.

What to take on board

- Mini toothbrush and toothpaste – there's nothing worse than fuzzy-feeling teeth!

- Mini deodorant – well, for obvious reasons.

- Mini pack of wipes – to freshen up (you know my thoughts on using them on your face so I'll say no more!).

- Socks – to keep your tootsies warm, the fluffier the better.

- Face mask – ideally, when flying wear no make-up. Your skin can get so dehydrated flying. I usually tan my face gradually on the days leading up to a flight (so at least I don't look like a ghost) then while on board I use a mask. **Glam Glows** hydrating mask is ideal as it's clear and you can leave it on as long as you like. If you do want to wear make-up, maybe just stay away from the heavy foundation and just use a tinted moisturizer, mascara and lip balm.

- Handcream – to help stop them drying out.

- Earphones – for music.

- Notebook and pen – I love scheming and dreaming while flying, and writing down my plans so I don't forget them.

*In between goals
is a thing called 'Life'
that has to be lived
and enjoyed.*

Sid Caesar

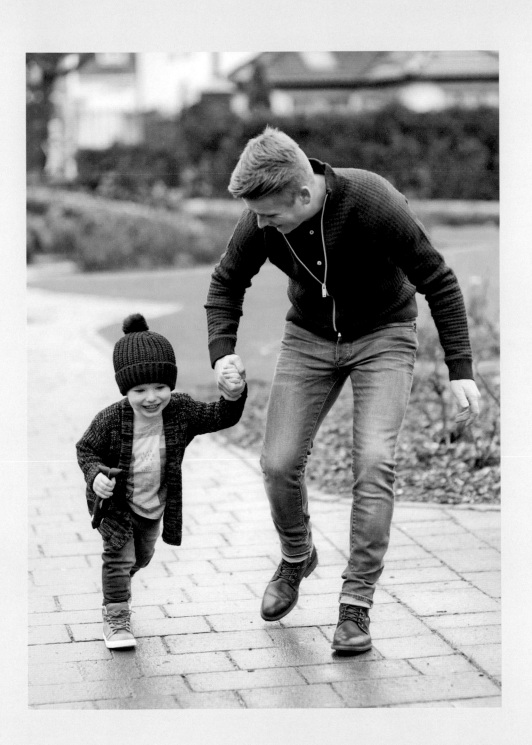

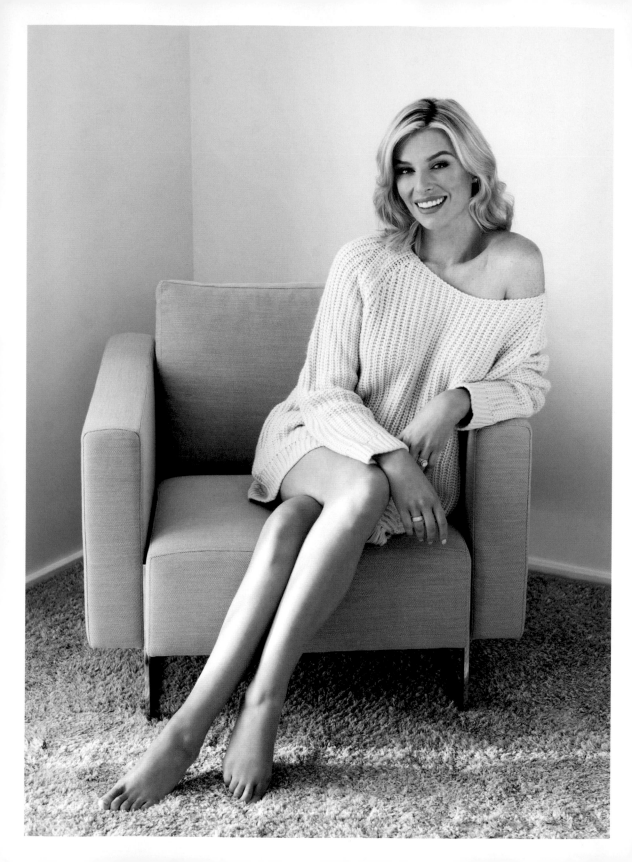

BE GOOD TO YOURSELF

I really hope you've enjoyed reading my book as much as I've enjoyed writing it. Hopefully, you'll take bits and pieces from it when you need it or re-read the book every now and then when you're looking for some ideas or inspiration.

So much of this book has been inspired by the emails I get every day at pippa.ie and all the women I meet at my Fashion Factories. They are the reason I wanted to write the book and their feedback and comments have really helped me to decide what to include in it.

Meeting so many people over the years, it's also struck me that we all seem to lead such hectic lives. I'm certainly on the go all the time and constantly moving on to the next thing. Sometimes we put a lot of pressure on ourselves, so I wanted the book also to help people readdress the balance a bit, to zone out of their everyday busy lives to enjoy a bit of 'me' time.

When my mum passed away so suddenly, it really stopped me in my tracks. At the time, I remember a friend telling me to be good to myself, a simple piece of advice that has stayed with me. It's so important to look after yourself, whatever you're going through in life.

*Every experience,
no matter how bad it
seems, holds within it
a blessing of some kind.
The goal is to find it.*

Buddha

So, take some time out – go for a walk, go to the hairdressers, leave the kids with family, meet a friend for a coffee or have that pamper night you've been promising yourself. It's not being selfish, it's the opposite as making time for yourself and recharging the batteries is going to make you a better person in the long run. Your kids will survive and the house can stay untidy for a little while longer!

Go easy on yourself and stop trying to be a superwoman. You can't be amazing at everything, nor can you do everything all at once. Focus on one thing at a time. I make notes and tick them off one by one now instead of trying to do five tasks at once. If you're in the office, be in the office. If you're at home cooking dinner and chatting to your kids, do it wholeheartedly. Let your mind be present in the moment.

And when life gets too overwhelming and you feel you can't cope – this happens to all of us! – just stop. Breathe. Switch off from the world of social media and emails and just be with your friends or family.

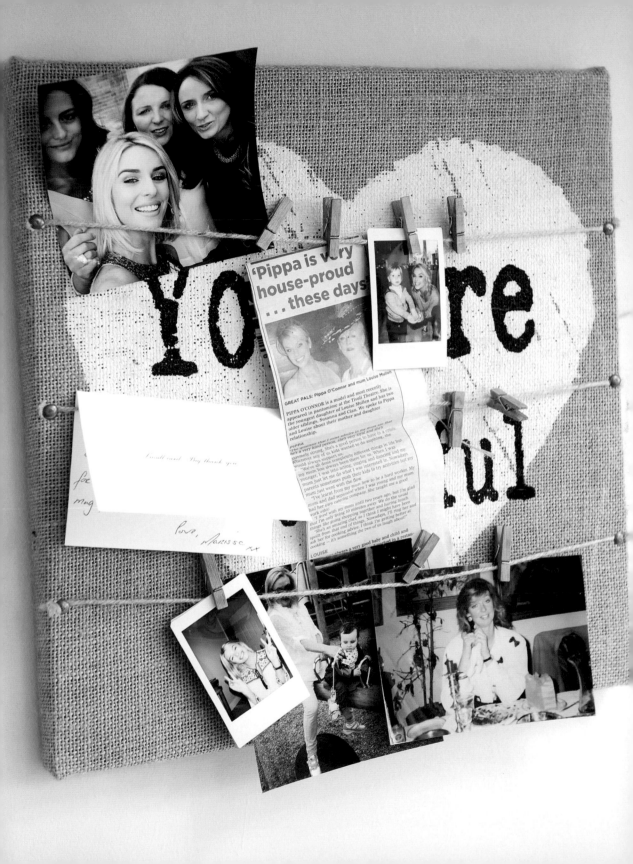

Ultimately your health and wellbeing is the most important thing you can have so it's vital you think about what's going on in your mind and body. I now know when that horrible anxious feeling is coming upon me – I nip it in the bud by stopping what I'm doing. Talking to my husband or a friend, followed by a hot bath and early night – that usually does the trick.

Something else that losing my mother and growing older has taught me is to give everything my best shot and not to be scared of failure. I've tried loads of things over the years that have failed and heard plenty of no's but if I hadn't tried I'd never have known. Nothing great is ever going to happen if you let fear dictate your life. Try not to worry what other people think about you, and in fact the less you care, the happier you'll be – this is so true!

Also, don't waste your time envying other people. That person who appears to have it all, I assure you, doesn't. Everyone faces their own battles and challenges and we all have different goals in life. Just treat everyone with kindness and do what works for you.

Trust that everything in life will work out just the way it's supposed to, at the right time. I really believe that positivity is the key to living happily. Even when things go horribly wrong try to see the positive in every situation. Your mind is a powerful thing and when you fill it with positive thoughts, your life will begin to change. Your thoughts become your reality if you just believe it enough.

If you want to live beautifully, look after your body *and* your mind – and be good to yourself!

Much love
Pippa x

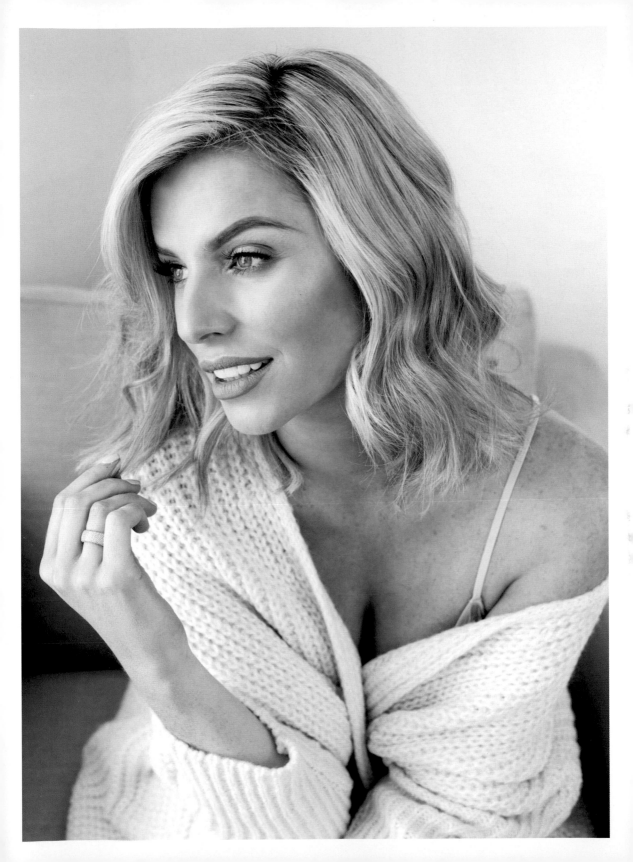

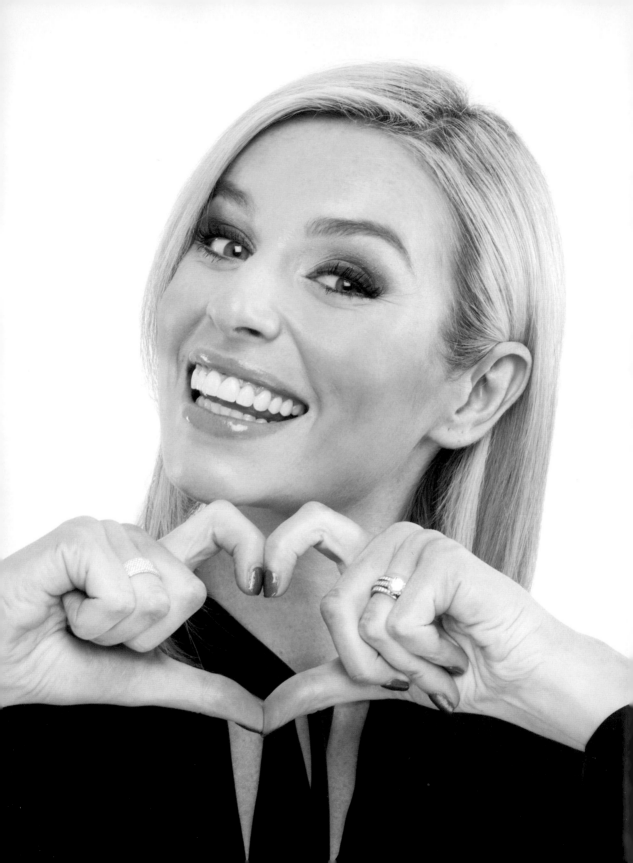

THANK YOU!

There's so many people I want to thank for helping me complete my first book.

First, Claire Pelly at Penguin – thank you for seeing something in me and introducing me to the wonderful Penguin team. I'm still embarrassed that I cried at our first meeting! If it wasn't for you contacting me I think I would have put my dream of writing a book on the long finger.

To Michael McLoughlin and Patricia Deevy at Penguin. Thank you for giving me free rein and allowing me to write what I wanted, but mostly thank you for taking a chance on me.

To Emma Marriott and Annabel Wright, thank you for advising and guiding me throughout my book journey. To be honest I had absolutely no idea how difficult and time-consuming it would be, which was probably a good thing in hindsight; ignorance was bliss on this occasion. So thank you both for your guidance, professionalism and patience with me. To designer Dan Newman, thank you for your incredible input. And thanks to the extended Penguin team for your hard work and support.

Now that this book is complete, it's the greatest feeling in the world. All those hours of hard work I put into it have been so worthwhile – I'm so excited and thrilled to be sharing my thoughts and passions with everyone.

I have lots of other people who helped get me to this stage:

Thank you to Jenny and Alan Taaffe and the team of iZest marketing for helping me and advising me every step of the way. Not just on the book but with all things pippa.ie.

To Freda, thank you for your advice and help – in more ways than one!

To Niamh Doherty, my right-hand woman in pippa.ie – thank you for keeping our ship afloat on weeks that I was absent, you're a little gem!

To my extended family and friends for simply being there for me – I love you all.

To my sister Susanna (Susu), thank you for everything! For telling me how it is, for looking out for me, for encouraging me on days when I had little energy and for not only being the best big sister but for acting as my mum too!

To my beautiful Ollie – although you have no idea what an impact being your mummy has been for me. I owe so much to you. You've given me the confidence and drive to believe in myself and just to let go and give it my best shot. After all, if I can do the most important job of all, being a mother – I can do anything!

To my readers and followers of pippa.ie – thank you so so much for your loyalty and support over the past three years. Thank you for always being so kind and encouraging. Thank you for believing in me. I've had the pleasure of meeting so many of you through my Fashion Factories and hopefully I'll meet many more of you at my book signings and other endeavours – but to those I've never met but who class me as a friend thank you! Because if it wasn't for all of you and your continued interest I

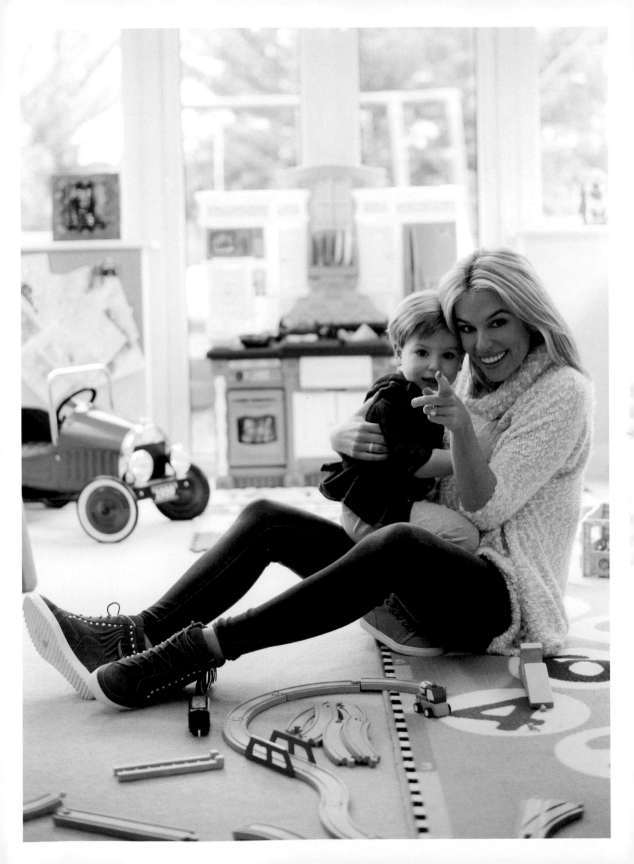

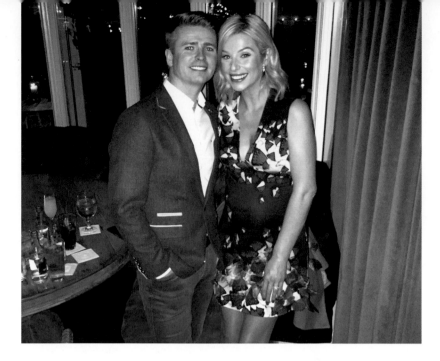

wouldn't be doing what I'm doing and certainly wouldn't be writing this book. Your amazing comments and kindness are what makes me want to do more all of the time. I'm so grateful for every single one of you.

Finally to my husband Brian – my biggest supporter and encourager of all. People often say to me: 'Wow, you're always on the go and so busy, how do you do it all?' I'm no superwoman, that's for sure – I'm just incredibly lucky to have wonderful people around me that I can lean on. It would be impossible for me to pursue my dreams without the help of my husband. Thank you especially for giving me the time to write this book, for acting as both Mummy and Daddy on many an occasion and not only did you not once complain but you also kept me going and focused. Nothing is ever a problem when you're around – you're kind and generous to a fault, which is why I love you so much! Thank you from the bottom of my heart.

Best wishes,
Pippa O'Connor Ormond

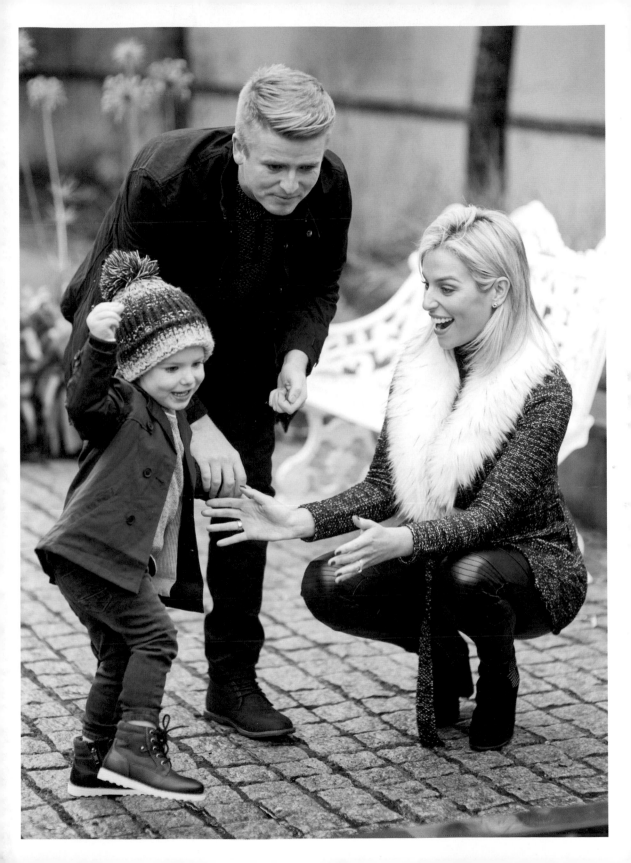

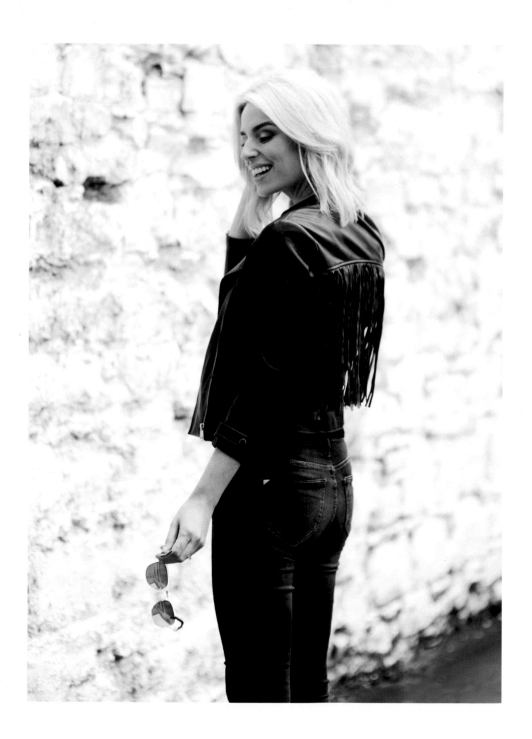